The Pegging Book

Also by Cooper S. Beckett

Osgood as Gone:
The Spectral Inspector, Book 1 (2019)

Osgood Riddance:
The Spectral Inspector, Book 2 (2019)

Approaching the Swingularity:
Tales of Swinging & Polyamory in Paradise (2017)

A Life Less Monogamous:
A Novel About Swinging (2016)

My Life on the Swingset:
Adventures in Swinging & Polyamory (2015)

The Pegging Book

A Complete Guide to Anal Sex with a Strap-On Dildo

Cooper S. Beckett and Lyndzi Miller

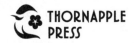

THORNAPPLE PRESS

The Pegging Book
A Complete Guide to Anal Sex with a Strap-On Dildo

Thornapple Press
300–722 Cormorant Street
Victoria, BC V8W 1P8 Canada
press@thornapplepress.ca

Thornapple Press (formerly Thorntree Press) is a brand
of Talk Science to Me Communications Inc. Our business
offices are located in the traditional, ancestral and unceded
territories of the ləkʷəŋən and W̱SÁNEĆ peoples.

Cover photo/illustration ©2022 by ksandrphoto
Cover design by Brianna Harden
Interior design by Jeff Werner
Interior illustrations by Cooper S. Beckett
Substantive editing by Andrea Zanin
Copy-editing by Hazel Boydell
Proofreading by Heather van der Hoop
Indexing by Maria Hypponen

Library and Archives Canada Cataloguing in Publication
  Title: The pegging book : a complete guide to anal sex with a
    strap-on dildo / Cooper S. Beckett and Lyndzi Miller.
  Names: Beckett, Cooper S., author. | Miller, Lyndzi, author.
  Description: Includes index.
  Identifiers:
    Canadiana (print) 20220274428 | Canadiana (ebook) 20220274460 |
    ISBN 9781778242090 (softcover) | ISBN 9781990869020 (PDF) |
    ISBN 9781990869006 (EPUB) | ISBN 9781990869013 (Kindle)
  Subjects: LCSH: Strap-on sex. | LCSH: Anal sex.
  Classification: LCC HQ31.5.D55 B43 2022 | DDC 306.77—dc23

10 9 8 7 6 5 4 3 2 1

Printed in the United States of America.

To our constellations

Contents

Acknowledgments

Cooper would like to thank his constellation: Elle and Wren, the Life on the Swingset crew; Ginger and Dylan; Tristan Taormino for promising him that prostate orgasms were possible; and Keeley for proving it.

Lyndzi would like to thank her husband, Rob, for supporting her in anything she sets her mind to, and The Tool Shed staff for helping her become a better sexual health educator and human.

They both would like to thank Ruby Ryder for her long-running discussion and celebration of the act of pegging on her *Pegging Paradise* podcast.

And finally, they'd like to thank each other for being wonderfully filthy pegging perverts.

Foreword:
Welcome to the Revolution

Tristan Taormino
Author of *The Ultimate Guide to Anal Sex for Women* and other books, sex educator, and creator of Sex Educator Boot Camp

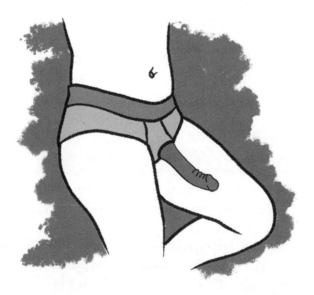

All big changes of the world come from words.
—Marjane Satrapi

In 2001, famed sex columnist Dan Savage ran a contest for his readers to come up with a new term to describe strap-on anal penetration in which women are the givers and men the receivers. Dan reported the most popular one that people submitted, and a new word was coined: pegging. The fact that a word exists for this activity is significant in and of itself. Naming something acknowledges its existence in our society, making it real, visible, and readable. It creates a shorthand for what is otherwise a clunky series of explanatory words. It gives people a way to express their desire and be understood based on shared meaning. It is powerful when there is a name for what we do.

The basic components of pegging—women doing the fucking and men getting fucked—make gender integral to the equation. The term conveys the radical possibilities of playing with, shifting, or upending gender roles in the context of sex. (When I use the words woman and man, I mean everyone who is a woman or a man regardless of their bodies, genitals, or what's on their birth certificates). Pegging is also about power: It reveals the power inherent in different roles and preconceived notions about who is and is not powerful. It takes the supposedly stable connection between gender and who gets to penetrate whom and exposes it as a lot more fluid than traditional heterosexuality would have us believe. Pegging is a game changer in both theory and practice.

Pegging doesn't just expand the language of sex; it expands the possibilities. For far too long, the cock has been marked as the site of sexual pleasure, the only game in town, the one spot you focus on. That notion oversimplifies the sexuality of penis and prostate owners and limits their ability to imagine and experience other erogenous zones, forms of stimulation, and types of orgasms. It confines pleasure to a narrow definition and robs people with dicks of the real complexity of their desires and fantasies. In the simplest terms, pegging opens up the body's erotic landscape and adds another savory/sweet treat to the menu.

I remember a coaching call I had with a straight, seventy-five-year-old retired businessman who worked in the medical industry. When I asked him about his sex life, he said, "My sex life has been going strong since my twenties and never slowed down. But I discovered anal play early on, so when my erections stopped working the way they usually did, it didn't deter me. A lot of my friends were panicked, getting scrips for Viagra, and bemoaning the lack of sexual pleasure in their lives. I just pivoted to focus on anal and the party kept going!"

Anal play and pegging do give you more options for pleasure. And getting fucked in the ass can be anything you want it to be. I've done pegging scenes that were gentle and loving, fun and carefree, degrading and humiliating, fast and furious, dominant and submissive. There is no one way to peg or be pegged. On a deeper level, to displace the cock from being at the center of sex, even temporarily, is revolutionary. It destabilizes what heterosexual sex is supposed to be. Come for the radical shift in heterosexuality, stay for the mind-bending orgasms!

The word pegging didn't exist when I began writing the first edition of *The Ultimate Guide to Anal Sex for Women* in 1997. Of course, people were pegging, so I wrote about the activity in my book; there is even an original illustration by underground artist Fish depicting this kind of strap-on sex, but very few people were talking about it publicly. Folks had trouble saying "anal sex" out loud back then. So much has changed in the past twenty-five years, and today mainstream media outlets like *Cosmopolitan* and *Men's Health* don't blink an eye at running features on anal toys for men, prostate stimulation, and pegging. *Esquire* has published an article titled "Why All Men Should Try Pegging (And How to Do It Properly)." Read that again, and marvel at the evolution of sexual norms.

Whenever more people are exposed to the concept of pegging, it's a good thing, although arguably when pegging had one of its biggest viral moments, it wasn't necessarily under ideal circumstances. Public discussions about pegging reached a fever pitch after the 2021 Met Gala, an event known for pushing the limits of avant-garde fashion. Model Cara Delevingne wore a white top—a cross between a vest and a large bib with multiple straps on each side where the skin of her torso peeked out. It read PEG THE PATRIARCHY in red block letters. People were frantically Googling. Those of us in sex-positive communities recognized the phrase immediately. It was coined in 2015 by Toronto-based sex educator Luna Matatas (who trademarked it in Canada in 2018), and we already owned t-shirts from her with "Peg the Patriarchy" in hot pink letters on them. The mainstream loves to invent or discover "new" things that people on the margins have been saying and doing for years.

In the press, Delevingne had the opportunity to discuss the origins of the phrase and uplift the work of a woman of color, but she didn't—another stark example of an industry co-opting the work of an independent artist. Twitter spread the word about Matatas and the origins of the phrase, but no acknowledgment or royalty checks were forthcoming from Delevingne or Christian Dior. Social media caught fire about it as both a fashion statement and a literal statement with hot takes like:

Yes! Let's do EXACTLY that. —@EmBello9

Cara Delevingne is breaking the internet with this viral message at the [Met Gala] #Feminism #WomensRights #peggingwife #FeministResponse —@NYN_News

Pegging is very pleasurable. I don't think
that pleasure is what you want to give
the patriarchy. —@dearnonnatives

Promoting the idea a man taking a woman's
dick in his ass necessarily involves being
overthrown, overpowered, annihilated,
destroyed, abolished, embarrassed, humiliated,
discomfited, or otherwise shamed as men
traditionally shame women is actually exactly
the work of patriarchy. —@9billiontigers

As someone who wears the message emblazoned
on my own chest and feels a sense of clarity about
what it means, I was surprised at so many alternate
readings. Matatas herself explained her intention
behind the phrase:

I wanted to start these conversations about the ways
in which equity is connected to our empowerment
but also our erotic side. We play a lot with fantasy
and power and we can use those metaphors in
our social activism. It really is a metaphor. Pegging
is a fantasy about anal penetration. But it's not
so much about anal sex. It's not so much about
cis-men. Because patriarchy has no gender. It's
a system and it affects everybody. We're all in a
position of either power or subservience under

> patriarchy. Which doesn't work for anybody.
> So "peg the patriarchy" is kind of saying, Let's
> subvert this. Let's not obey and be subservient.

There is a case to be made that "Peg the Patriarchy" is a playful middle finger, in the form of a dildo up the ass of a system of oppression, but I think it's more complicated than that. I read it in several ways. If "peg" is a stand-in for "fuck," it's a word with multiple meanings and contexts, from the sexual ("I want to fuck you") to the aggressive ("Fuck you!"). So, if we take it as a form of "fuck the patriarchy," we're fucking the institutionalized oppression of women and femmes in a decidedly queer, non-normative way, which itself is subversive. The phrase can also be translated as: let's turn the patriarchy on its head the way pegging turns the very notion of what "straight" sex is on its head. Or: let's dismantle the patriarchy the way pegging dismantles heterocentric sex. Also: let's strap on a symbolic form of the patriarchy along with the power it wields. Let's infiltrate the patriarchy and get inside a place where we've been told we don't belong, the way a slick dildo slips inside another taboo and off-limits space. Let's revel when the patriarchy surrenders its soft, pink, vulnerable opening to a woman, which goes against what the patriarchy is supposed to be and do. I could go on. Language is important. Words and their meanings matter. Especially when it comes to sexuality.

The patriarchy belongs in a discussion about pegging because the personal is political and sex is both a private intimacy and a political act. Sex is especially politicized when how we fuck falls outside the lines of narrow heterocentric categories, challenging norms, defying categorization, and screwing with people's beliefs. And nothing says "look over here, I am outside that box" like pegging! It is a powerful symbol in the language of fucking because the roles of the penetrator and the penetrated can be played by anyone. Suddenly all bets are off and everything you were taught about sex is wrong! As quickly as you can buckle a few straps, pegging dismantles the man-woman-penis-vagina foundation of heterosexual sex. Central ideas that heteronormativity holds dear begin to fall away, especially those about bodies, genitals, what you can and can't do with them, and how they bring us pleasure.

It's fascinating that a word rooted in gender roles actually has the power to obliterate and transcend gender. Everyone has an asshole, so anyone can peg and get pegged.

In this moment, pegging might seem old-fashioned to some since it relies on the gender binary. Language is dynamic and ever changing, and the language of gender has dramatically shifted in the last two decades. People have been resisting two narrow choices since the beginning of time, as well as contesting, challenging, and redefining "woman" and "man." What has changed is that the words we use have evolved to recognize how the gender binary has been stretched, smashed, and re-fashioned. How does pegging's original meaning hold up? What about when a nonbinary person does a transmasculine guy in the ass with a strap-on? How about someone genderqueer strapping it on to penetrate their genderfluid lover's butt? I want to harness all the possibilities that pegging has to offer, but I do not wish to ignore, exclude, or erase folks for whom "man" and "woman" don't represent their gender: people who are both, neither, or somewhere on or off the gender spectrum.

But let's not throw out all the clean dildos with the soapy water just yet. Our world adapted to pegging once, and I believe strongly that pegging can adapt to our world. Perhaps it will adapt to incorporate the play between masculine and feminine (also a binary, I know). Or it will replace words like buttfuck (which now means a penis, itself defined in narrow ways, in an ass), bugger (the old-school word that originated in England), or sodomize (too clinical and foreboding, if you ask me). The point is that pegging emerged in a specific historical context and gave millions of people a way to name their sex. In the process, it shattered old ideas about sex roles, who can do what, and the scope of all the perverse pleasures in which we can partake. It redefined sexuality for all genders.

You're about to get lots of great information about pegging from Cooper and Lyndzi, two fantastic sex educators with a wealth of knowledge about it and experience doing it. They've done a thoughtful, thorough job of exploring all the nuance and complexity (and fun) this kind of sex has to offer, and they do it in a way that's sex-positive, holistic, and very accessible, like talking to a couple of friends who also happen to be experts. Is pegging your favorite pastime? Has pegging unlocked new worlds of eroticism for you? Has pegging changed the way you think about sex and gender? Did you pick up this book because you are interested but haven't yet tried it? Whoever you are, welcome to the revolution. It all starts here.

Introduction:
New Book, Who Dis?

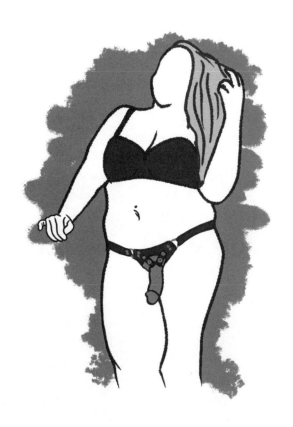

We, your authors, Lyndzi and Cooper, are not doctors, and thus the advice in this book is for novelty purposes only. As such, the content within, unless otherwise cited, is based upon our personal opinions and understanding of bodily functions, through conversation, observation, or personal exploration. What we're saying is, don't take our word as gospel, always watch out for your health, use only toys with flared bases, and maybe consult a doctor if you're going to use a dildo thicker than your forearm.

Just a thought.

"If you're not doctors, then who are you?" you ask.

We're self-styled educators. We don't have silly things like degrees or credentials (can you imagine if one could get a PhD in pegging?), but we do have a wealth of experience. What people used to call street smarts. Although our very specific fields of knowledge, namely sexuality and the vast plethora of implements one can use to pleasure themselves and others, may not get us too far on the mean streets of any major metropolitan area, they have proved useful to many.

Many years ago, we began teaching a class at Milwaukee's The Tool Shed: An Erotic Boutique, an adult toy store and part of a revolution of feminist, queer, and/or women-run stores clapping back at the old creepy dungeons of jelly dildos with masturbation booths in the back. Our class, titled "Take It Like a Man," was continually sold out and rerun time after time. Each time we'd get to the end and begin talking about resources for more information about this wacky thing called "pegging," we'd realize that aside from a couple of older books (including an excellent one by our foreword mistress Tristan Taormino) that focused on a more generalized conception of anal sex, there just *wasn't* a book about pegging. At the end of each class we would say: "Maybe we should write one."

Suddenly a pandemic appeared and amid the awful whole apocalypse thing, we thought this was a time where we might actually be able to focus and write such a book.

"Maybe you should write this, maybe you did teach the class, but who *are* you?"

Alright, alright. Lyndzi Miller cut her teeth in the trenches themselves, working at The Tool Shed for over a decade, answering questions, recommending products, and sharing knowledge accumulated, researched, and gathered from her personal life. Cooper S. Beckett is a journeyman writer and creator who co-started a podcast about swinging that ballooned way beyond his expectations and led to him writing a memoir and two novels about non-monogamy and sexuality. In between those projects, he took time to do what he hesitated to call "teaching" at conferences all around the world, including at The Tool Shed in Milwaukee.

On top of those credentials? Well, we both really enjoy pegging! And we think we can help you enjoy it, too. In addition to reading this book, we encourage you to visit thepeggingbook.com/bonus, where you'll find worksheets to download and additional resources.

Content Notes

Because the concept of pegging is rather heterocentric and gendered culturally (i.e., a non-penis-haver anally penetrating a penis-haver with a strap-on/harnessed dildo), we will be using a lot of heterocentric language. That said, we want to acknowledge that not all penis-havers are men, not all men have penises or prostates, not all vulva-havers are women, and not all women have vulvas or G-spots. We do our best to use inclusive language but recognize that sometimes the inclusive language is less clear.

We also use profanity—a fucking lot, in fact—as it's just more fun to talk about sex using words like fucker and fuckee. Because of our propensity for profanity, we will alternate the words we use for things seemingly at random. One paragraph it'll be a penis, another it'll be a dick, still another a cock. But we can tell you one thing for sure: we will NEVER refer to anything except the vaginal canal as a vagina. The rest is the vulva, people. C'mon!

We will also endeavor to define our terms early and often, so we hope to cover all the sexy verbiage and pegging jargon along the way.

Throughout the body of this book, we will use "we" to refer to ourselves, the authors. Occasionally, we will insert sections with our personal recollections in the first person. Don't worry, we'll tell you when. Otherwise, these thoughts, opinions, plans, and ideas belong to both of us.

We also reached out to thousands of couples, triads, and singles to ask their thoughts on pegging, and for any questions they might have, and have used their questions and thoughts to help craft the book you have in front of you.

One more note. It's a world of flux out there, isn't it? We don't suppose that will ever *truly* change, but we can say that it's no stretch to assume that some people picking up this book think very differently than we do, be it religiously, politically, or progressively. Does that matter, really, though?

If we're on the same page with a desire for a safe and consensual sex act, isn't that all that matters? Well, it should be, probably, but we're not going to sit here and sugarcoat the fact that both of us are pretty hard-core liberals, and we don't hide those views in the pages that follow. You can be certain that there's going to be nothing but enthusiastic support for sex workers, the rights of the LGBTQIA+ community, and others in this book.

Why couldn't we keep that stuff out of here? Well, sex is political. Pegging itself could be considered a radical act. It doesn't have to be, and nothing that follows will point out groups or ethos that somehow should bar you from participating in pegging or enjoying the act. We invite all on this journey.

So, with all that behind us, allow us to set the mood. (Using second-person prose, no less!)

You're sitting on the back patio of a delightfully divey bar that has an outdoor firepit. We, Cooper and Lyndzi, sit across from you. We share a drink, we make merry. Then, summoning your courage, you cautiously lean across to where we sit and ask us the big question, the one we're going to hit in our first chapter: "What is pegging?"

We laugh, not in a mocking way, but because we love your question and are absolutely thrilled to be given the opportunity to answer it. After glancing around the patio to see who's in earshot (and assess if those who might hear are also "cool"), we let smiles cross our faces and begin to tell you about one of the coolest and sexiest of sex acts.

What Is Pegging?

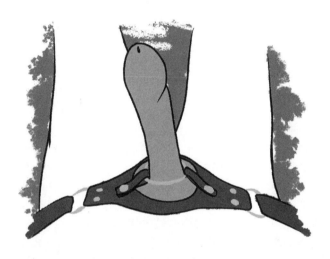

In the beginning, there was no name for it.

The act was lumped in with general anal sex and general strap-on sex. But perhaps seeing a hole that needed filling, *Savage Lovecast* held a contest to name the act. When the dust had settled, the word was clear, and the world had changed.

peg • ging (verb): A sex act in which a woman penetrates a man, anally, with a strap-on dildo

Unlike most sex acts named literally, clinically, or organically (from ten-year-olds in the streets bragging about doing things of which they actually have no concept), pegging was dubbed, and thus a whole new porn category was officially born.

The question has to be asked: "Why does pegging get perhaps the most specific and heterocentric definition of all the sex acts?" Well, traditionally, if you're a man having anal sex with another man, that's already categorized as anal sex. If you're a woman using a strap-on to fuck another woman, that's also already categorized as strap-on sex. And if you're a man fucking a woman in the ass…guess what, anal sex again, or if we want to go back to our giggly twelve-year-old brains, buttfucking. And can we all agree that buttfucking just sounds weirdly natural in a way that assfucking doesn't?

While we'll agree that pegging doesn't really need its own term, and should rightly be slotted into the strap-on sex category, a number of factors that surround it cause us to believe it worth keeping in its own category, at least for the time being. Namely, there's so much stigma around the act and the idea of men…well…taking it like a man and receiving anal stimulation, that it sort of needs the spotlight to be shined on it. Someday the world may be ready to welcome pegging into other categories, but for now we need a term that's very obvious and not avoiding what we're talking about. In our manly man, patriarchal society, it's unfortunately a common thought that being a "receiver" of sex (the "fucked" rather than the "fucker") and, god forbid, letting *anything* in through the out door makes a man somehow less of a man.

Combining this often-homophobic stigma with a general fear of discussing anything sexual that we don't quite understand or haven't tried, it's a tall order to share information about pegging. In writing this book, in fact, we've been struggling with a certain giant online retailer, asking it to explain to us why it has slotted our educational (at least edu-tainment) book about pegging into the "adult" category while it lets others, including erotica, roam free.

That's why we have taught our pegging class over and over throughout the years, always with standing room only. People want to know, but are afraid to ask. We understand the fear, of course—we were not always the titans of sex education we hope people see us as. No one knows anything, we like to say, until we know.

So often, though, the question is asked, of us, of others, always in a hushed, breathy whisper: "We've been thinking about getting into...pegging. Do you know what that is?"

At The Tool Shed boutique, Lyndzi always notices visible relief in the eyes of these customers. She leads them to the harness rack and to the shelves upon shelves of friendly and unthreatening brightly colored dildos.

Being able to talk about your sexual fantasies to your partner is hard enough, but going out into the world to attempt to make this happen, into an intimidating sex toy store (even one as cute and chill as The Tool Shed), and admitting to a total stranger that you want to be fucked in the ass by your partner or want to fuck your partner in the ass, can be incredibly scary. *What if they think I'm gay? What if they think I'm sick and depraved? What if they think my sexual desires are wrong or shameful? Worse yet, what if they're right?*

Do not fret, friend. Let us be your helpful harness and dildo fairies. Through this magical little book, we can teach you the sexy skill and, dare I say, art of pegging.

Why Call It Pegging?

Why someone should call it "strap-on sex" versus "pegging" or vice versa is a common question asked in sex-positive spaces. Let's get into it! First though, we're going to throw a couple words at you that you may be unfamiliar with, so here are a few definitions:

Heterocentrism: the commonly held, societally enforced belief that heterosexual activities are better than LGBTQIA+ activities (or those activities without a gender assigned to them at all), and the belief that hetero things are considered the only "normal" or "true" way.

Cis: shorthand for someone who was assigned a certain gender at birth and who agrees with that assessment (e.g., When I was born, I came out of the womb with a vulva and because of that, the doctor and my parents called me a girl. Growing up, I agreed with that, and I now identify as a woman, so I am cis or cisgender).

Trans: shorthand for someone who was assigned a certain gender at birth and who does not agree with that assessment (e.g., I was born with a penis so the doctor and my parents called me a boy. Growing up, I came to realize that I did not agree with this assumption and now identify as a woman, so I am a trans woman (or just a woman, no clarifier needed, because, simply put, trans women are women).

Cishet: a shorthand term for a cisgender, heterosexual person. Some folks have demonized the word because it makes them feel othered, which makes them feel uncomfortable, when they think what they are is the "norm" (literally that word up there, "heterocentrism," rearing its ugly head). What's normal, anyway, right? Identifying as cisgender and telling people your pronouns just normalizes clarifying these things for the rest of the world and is a good, positive thing to do overall.

Cissexism: much like heterocentrism, this is the belief that cisgender folks are "normal" or "better" than trans folks. It's also the assumption that everyone is cis until stated otherwise and treating trans people like only they need to disclose their pronouns because we should all be able to assume what pronouns to use based on looks. This just isn't based in reality and erases the existence of nonbinary folks (people who don't identify as men or women).

When talking about pegging as an act "reserved" for heterosexual couples, there are a lot of folks who get left out of the equation who can still use all of the information held here in these pages. Talking about prostates as if all men have them is just inaccurate. Some men have had their prostates removed due to cancer and some were never born with them to begin with (like trans men). If you think about pegging as an act between a man and a woman, that doesn't necessarily exclude trans folks (because, again, trans women are women and trans men are men, yo). Though if you make it specific to penis- and vulva- havers, that also doesn't really work, since women, both trans and cis, can peg men, both trans and cis, regardless of genitals. Even saying that pegging is for heterosexual couples leaves out bisexual and queer identifying couples.

Is your head spinning yet? It's okay, this is a lot of information.

We spoke to polyamorist writer, activist, sex worker, porn star, and generally amazing human Andre Shakti about this concern. "I'm seeing much more of a conflation of the terms strap-on sex and pegging," she said.

In sex-positive spaces, most folks like labels to clarify acts, behaviors, identities, whatever. Labels help, but when they're redundant or the label itself is deemed harmful, they're usually cast aside. Pegging is one of those terms that because it is ultimately strap-on sex, is seen as redundant, especially in queer communities where strap-ons hang from every closet door and dildos are used as artistic room decor.

"As you and I know," Shakti stated, "pegging was basically created...to describe, very literally, what is strap-on sex, just between two heterosexual, cisgender-identified individuals. The more I teach about it, the more I hear people, including heterocentric or heterosexual couples, just calling it plain old 'strap-on sex,' which I think honestly is a much more sex-positive way of addressing it, just because I don't think it's necessary for a separate term to exist just because we're speaking about a different body."

The reality of the situation is, for folks who aren't in the sex-positive community—which is unfortunately most of the world—there's still a lot of stigma, mystery, and curiosity surrounding strap-on sex, especially between a heterosexual couple. Strap-on sex in the queer and lesbian communities is pretty old hat at this point—they have that down to a science.

As it stands now, for those cishet couples and anyone else interested in anal sex or strap-on play, we have written this book. Eventually, we hope the world becomes a more sexually aware, more sex-positive place in general. We hope that in the future, terms like pegging might not be necessary at all. Gendered terms will be considered passé, maybe even politically incorrect. Maybe in the future, everyone will consider pegging to be boring and commonplace. "Oh, you pegged your husband last night? Who cares, I jigsawed a literal stranger in the street last night. Get with the program, TK421," some futuristic twenty-something will sneer at her boring, cishet friend.

We can dream.

Until then, we'd like to talk about strap-on sex, about anal sex, and about pegging.

Other Verbiage

Since we're already defining terms, we thought we might want to get a bunch of other ones out of the way.

Alright, so, as we discussed, pegging is the fucking of someone else in the ass with a strap-on dildo, and phrased that way so we're going gender-neutral. A **strap-on dildo** is an often and most safely silicone phallus that is attached to the wearer with a **harness** that can come in many styles (leather straps, underoos, you name it) and that holds the dildo in place. Many will sell you stories of the **strapless strap-on**, which is usually just a dildo with an extra bit on the end to go up deep inside the pegger. If you have excellent **Kegel muscles** (your pelvic floor muscles—you can test them by stopping your pee mid-stream), you *may* be able to hold one of these bad boys in.

Some peggees, many of the **AMAB** type (Assigned Male at Birth), but not all, have **prostates**, which are glands that feel like a spongy walnut on the topside of the rectum. The prostate gives your cum some extra oomph fluid and also occasionally goes rogue and gets all cancery. If you own one of these and are on the more middle-to-late side of adulthood, please get yours checked. We will cheekily sometimes refer to the prostate as the **P-spot** to align it with the **AFAB** (Assigned Female at Birth) **G-spot** (Gräfenberg spot), which is the same spongy walnut shape on the topside of the vaginal canal. And wouldn't you know it, science pretends it doesn't exist even after a German man decided to name it after himself.

Another term for pegger and peggee may be **top** and **bottom**, words borrowed from the queer community; top usually means giver and bottom receiver. While we're addressing the vast spectrum of queer and the **LGBTQIA+** community (Lesbian Gay Bisexual Trans Queer Intersex Asexual +), it might be helpful to remind people again that **trans women** are women and **trans men** are men and **nonbinary** folk are what they are, and that may or may not change from mood to mood, day to day, both consciously and not.

Some abbreviations we use are **PIV** (penis in vagina) and **PIA** (penis in anus) and really those penises could be dildos too, so...you do you. **Salad tossing** is a, let's be honest, really weird term for **analingus**, which is licking the butthole. We've also heard "velvet fruitloop" used for the same activity, but that may have just been a dream.

Fisting shouldn't need an explanation, but so people don't go all Caligula on someone, it is not making a fist and shoving it inside another person, but *is* putting your whole damned hand in there. And that hand can either go in a pussy or (really!) a butt. **Fingering** there's some debate on, like we *know* it's fingering if your finger goes inside a vagina or asshole, but is it still fingering when the finger just plays outside and never moves in? We, and the world, may never know.

STDs used to be the way we talked about big scary sexually transmitted diseases. But then we realized that most of these things are very manageable and less debilitating than the flu, so to soften that language we shifted it to **STIs** for sexually transmitted infections. Most infections, like most STIs, are entirely treatable and not actually all that scary. Don't you feel better already?

Many will argue that **come** is the way to spell both the orgasm as well as the fluid it makes. Others will argue that **cum** is the one true way. We'll split the difference and declare: it's come when referring to the moment of orgasm ("I'm coming!") and cum when you're referring to the mess someone just made on your clean sheets ("You got cum everywhere!").

Lube can really be anything that makes the going slicker, encompassing the body-safe stuff that we talk about at length later in the book, including silicone, water-based, and oil-based products, as well as the body-iffy stuff like coconut oil, olive oil, and Crisco. And then there's the no, stop, don't do that stuff such as butter, hand lotion, shampoo, and spit. Spit is not lube, people. Just...just fucking stop.

We will detail more types of lube, harnesses, and dildos in the Best Tools for the Job section later.

Anatomy

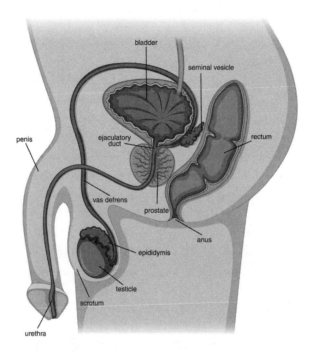

While we're sure you're all very familiar with bodies from paying extra-close attention in health class, we thought it might be worth getting to know the various faculties and functions of the naughty bits on your average penis-haver. So, with that, we bring you:

An Owner's Guide to the Male Reproductive System

Congratulations! You've gone and gotten yourself a male reproductive system. Whether factory installed or aftermarket, it's going to be pretty much the same thing, so let's take a quick tour.

Starting on the left, there is the penis. From the factory it comes with a lovely little foreskin turtleneck that some folks see fit to remove on delivery. Whether it's there or not, you're perfectly normal either way.

Then there's your urethra. That's a sort of super-highway for the various liquids that are going to be flushed from your system from time to time. You'll see that one of its two forks goes directly to your bladder. This is where pee comes from. You've seen that, though, so we're not going to go much deeper into it. The other fork of the urethra heads into the factory deep inside called the seminal vesicle.

Enclosed in a fleshy sack called the scrotum that offers little to no protection from anything are the testicles. This is where the sperms come from. Sperms are wriggly little cells that want nothing more than to jam their heads into an egg and, we presume, are very disappointed when they wind up on some tits, in some hair, on a belly, in a throat, or in a couple of tissues that are unceremoniously deposited into the garbage.

These sperms move from the testicles into the epididymis and then travel up the vas deferens to the seminal vesicles, where the semen comes from. Semen is part of the sperm delivery service and gets very sticky if left out. Best to wipe off quickly.

When a launch is imminent, the prostate begins lubing the runway with prostatic fluid or pre-cum. Then, when the counter reaches zero (or sometimes earlier, no shame), the prostatic fluid and the semen combine to flume-ride the sperm to Valhalla. Massaging the prostate through the wall of the rectum will cause it to engorge, and as it surrounds the urethra, you may feel the need...the need to pee.

All the above talk may make you think that these organs were designed only for functional purposes, but that isn't true! Most of the things on this list are also used for fun (and sometimes profit—we stand with sex workers.)

The P-Spot vs. the G-Spot

We may sound like a broken record here, and for that we apologize, but it is worth reiterating before we go deep (phrasing) about the P-spot and the G-spot that we are not doctors, we do not have any advanced degrees, and we are only relaying what we've learned elsewhere or have conceptualized ourselves. Some of what follows will probably be at the very least up for debate. That said, the G-spot isn't even recognized as a thing at all by most doctors, so we're gonna proceed with the understood concept that there is, in fact, a G-spot, and it is, in fact, awesome, and those who would deny it are just jealous. Y'know, like any mature book on a subject would.

For most men, their entire experience with prostate stimulation can be summed up by that vague discussion on sitcoms where men of a certain age suck in a breath when the words "prostate exam" are uttered. There's much to unpack with that, including homophobia, the humor in the idea of things in your pooper, and the most pertinent fact that no, your prostate exam is not supposed to be pleasurable or sexy in any way. They're checking your prostate, most definitely not massaging or playing with it.

What we mean is, while it's not supposed to hurt, your doctor's not hoping you enjoy the prostate exam. And your doctor is also likely well aware of the range of thoughts that go through the minds of typical men when told "drop your pants and bend over." The societal notions go into overdrive and the doctor just wants to get this over with as quickly as possible so you, the receiver of one of the simplest yet most dreaded exams for men, don't think too hard about the fact that you have another human's finger in your ass.

As such, the exam is done in a matter of seconds. KY jelly on the fingers and take a breath! Poke. Done.

As those of us who enjoy prostate play can tell you, there's nothing fun about fast and pokey. So, in an effort to mitigate the tension and pain, the exam is done in a way that causes tension and pain, and the wheel in the sky keeps on turning. And if that's your only experience with or perception of prostate stimulation, why on earth would you ever want to do it? (If you think we're not about to answer that very question, then you haven't been paying attention.)

'Cuz (deep breath) the prostate and the G-spot are pretty much the same thing. And to illustrate this in a non-doctory way (because not doctors, remember), we have to go way back to the beginning.

Alright. In the beginning (individual life beginning, not universe beginning), we are all female in the womb. We know, gender is merely a construct and not all women have vulvae and vaginas, but for the sake of simplicity, literally all of us have the building blocks of those vulvae and vaginas and ovaries inside us. For a few weeks anyway, this is true. Then that bullying Y chromosome either gets its way, or doesn't, and the paths diverge.

We're only talking about small masses of tissue at this point, remember, but the divergent paths follow wonderfully parallel development. The same bits either become ovaries or descend and become testicles. Those testicles are then covered by fused labia. (Ever notice that weird seam that splits the ballsack? That's what we're talking about.) A bundle of nerves either concentrates itself as the clitoris or tries to get as far away from the body as possible and becomes the head of the penis.

Well, you say, that's a lot of talk about stuff that you profess to not know much about in the beginning of a chapter about G-spots and P-spots.

Like a certain old Jewish man played by Eddie Murphy would say: "Aha! Aha!"

See, the fact that we were all once female makes the prostate interesting. Well, to us it does, anyway. Cooper just loves to explanabrag this part.

Once upon a time he was having a threeway with a wonderful couple and enjoying himself very much, as one does. Well, he found himself kneeling at the bottom of their bed while they both lay on their backs, with fingers inside both the mister and the missus at the same time. As he did the power gesture (the "come here" gesture) with his fingers, Coop felt the same thing happen in both of them at once!

His prostate, which felt like a squishy walnut, began to engorge and grow, and at the same time, on the roof of her vaginal canal, another mass of tissue that felt like a squishy walnut began to engorge and grow. And these magical engorged masses, when expertly stimulated, managed to produce orgasmic waves in both of these wonderful humans.

Cooper may be a braggart, but he did get to experience something that, frankly, people rarely do. Society's stigma surrounding group sex, and around bisexual males, definitely puts a kibosh on this sort of "hands-on" experimentation. His observation is right though—in nearly the same spot, surrounding the urethras of both men and women, these masses of tissue behave in almost the exact same way.

When using that "come here" gesture that those of us who've chased a squirting orgasm in women have learned well, we can elicit a very similar response in men. Both produce very similar orgasms.

Thus, with that albeit limited and very non-scientific standard, we can make a few entirely unscientific assertions and observations. Both men and women have some tissue surrounding their urethras that, when stimulated in specific (and similar) ways, can produce some ecstatic release that we'd be hard-pressed not to call an orgasm.

We've also found both personally and in discussions with friends with both G-spots and P-spots that when this area is stimulated, all report a strong feeling of needing to pee. This is likely due to the engorged tissue surrounding the urethra and pressing on the bladder. This is also unfortunately what has caused so many to dismiss squirting orgasms as "just peeing."

It's not, and even if it was, fuck you. No orgasm is "just" anything.

So, why all this buildup? Well, because, as with the dismissal of the G-spot entirely, many dismiss the notion that the prostate is a gland that can provide pleasure.

If you already have experience with G-spots, then congratulations—you pretty much know how to play with a prostate. Both enjoy pressure and rubbing, and both need to be warmed up before they're gone at hard.

Plus, there's definitely some evidence that prostate stimulation and regular flushing of prostatic fluid (that is, milking, or just run of the mill jackin' it) can lead to better prostate health in the long run, but that's more of a discussion for our next section, in which we will again remind you that *we are not doctors*.

Why Pegging Is Awesome

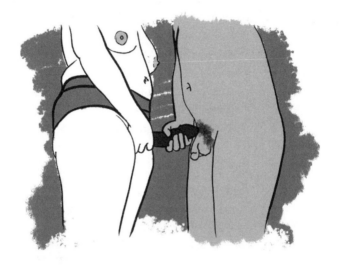

Benefits of Exploration

It's easy to become complacent in life, to sort of feel "finished" at a certain point, and not need to push outward in our ideas or practices. We do this because sometimes it can seem like it would take a lot of effort to try new things. But when one of the most frequently cited causes of conflict in a relationship is stagnant sex, the same-old, same-old, we really need to take control of the situation and work to continue our sexual growth throughout our entire lives. This isn't just necessary, but also fun.

Because pegging is rarely something that happens in a brand-new relationship (mainly because most people don't think of it, we reckon), the act is often a whole new area for most people to explore. We all know that exploration can feel scary, as the unknown brings a lot of fear.

What if I don't like it? What if they don't want to? What if it makes me gay? Well, let's get that last one right out of the way, as there's really no room for ambiguity here.

What If It Makes Me Gay?

Pegging will not make you gay! *Nothing* will *make* you gay!

Men seem to worry about this possibility more than anything in the world, and frankly, we blame toxic societal influences. Dammit, Chandler!

But there's no question—you are either gay, straight, or somewhere in between, and no single act is going to change who you are. A caveat to this: of course, you may discover through exploration, experimentation, and experience that you are actually gay when you thought you were straight or bi. This realization could seem enlightening, or frightening, or life-changing. But it is just that—a realization. And that exploration, experimentation, and experience did *not* make you gay, or bi, or anything else, it just showed you something you didn't yet know about yourself.

Besides, if you're gay, wouldn't you want to know it? It seems like something that would be valuable for life going forward. But that's neither here nor there, because there is nothing gay about the butt. Unless enjoying yourself is gay! (It's not.)

The anus has so many nerve endings, and those with a prostate can experience such pleasure through anal play, that rejecting it out of hand because of what "society" might think (who's gonna tell them? Not us) is like deciding you're happy with only half of your potential enjoyment in action. If you knew you could possibly double it by bringing your butt online, why *wouldn't* you do it?

So, the butt's not gay. Now, let's attack the second part of that: getting buttfucked (teehee) is gay. Well, buddy, we gotta say, we can think of few things *less* gay than a man having sex with a woman. So, as long as you're getting pegged (see the earlier definition), it's safe to assume that what you're doing is decidedly not gay.

What you *are* doing, though, is waking your body up. You know that old saying that you use only 10 percent of your brain? Well, first, that's bullshit—you use all of your brain—but the typical male run-and-gun orgasm pattern uses only 10 percent of your sexuality.

There are so many areas to be brought online, and the anus and prostate are two amazing pleasure avenues to wake up.

Role Reversal: Understanding Different Points of View

Let's take a moment to speak directly to the men.

We're not saying that *you* do this, but some men are known to fuck, come, and go. For many, sex is a short thing. This is not a problem—believe us, quickies are awesome—but once the man has an orgasm, it's over. And the man usually goes elsewhere after that. Home. To sleep. To watch some big sportsball game. Again, we're not calling *you* out, dear reader.

The very nature of pegging slows things down. Sure, it can be a thrusting, rollicking good time, but it takes preparation and finesse, and especially that slide inside should be deliciously slow. So, men, putting yourself in the receiving position means you can experience something entirely new. You can find out what it's like to receive, to "bottom," to be penetrated.

This type of heteronormative role reversal (meaning the assumption that the couple in question is heterosexual) gives you a unique point of view on what your partner does and has experienced. Pegging receivers learn that just jamming a dick in the ass maybe isn't the best way to go about anal sex. Peggers get to learn what it's like to do the brunt of the work of thrusting (what workout dudes have to do!).

In the reality of sex, we all come to learn that real life just isn't porn. Porn is *The Fast and the Furious* franchise, and we're all just learning how to shift gears. No one should learn how to drive by watching *The Fast and the Furious*, and yet so much of our sexual education (maybe miseducation?) comes from porn.

And now we're gonna speak directly to the women (but you men can keep reading if you'd like. Also, anyone who doesn't identify with either male or female, feel free to read. You're awesome.)

Our society has done women a disservice, well many disservices, but we're going to focus on a specific sexual one. Folks socialized as women are taught to be pursued, to avoid being aggressive, to play coy, to be demure. Fuck that. Fuck *them*. Women are powerful, and a woman pegging is even more so, and it's about time ladies took the reins and stuck it to the man…so to speak. Be loud, be aggressive, fuck how you like to fuck.

Pegging is an opportunity to see through your partner's eyes, as they look up at you with that dick hanging between your legs. And speaking of that dick, go ahead and stroke it. Having seen many women put their first harnesses on and their first dildos between their legs, the spark of realization in their eyes is delightful. As silly as we may find it, we've all spent some time considering what it might look like or feel like to have genitals other than what we've been given. Revel in it, women.

Play with your dick!

What If I Don't Like It?

This is a question that many of us ask before trying anything new, because new can mean scary for lots of us. There's nothing wrong with this, and worrying about not liking something new is not inherently a bad thing. Many of us resist the unknown due to feeling ashamed of not liking something, or not being good at something in our past. All of us at some point have worried about doing something new that seemed scary, so please don't feel ashamed if this is one of your concerns.

But the big secret that no one really talks about is the best answer to that question. That it's *okay* if you try something and don't like it. Then you just don't do it again. We're all in control of our bodies, and every experience is an opportunity to put something into categories. These aren't official—they're just off the top of our heads:

* I loved that and I want to do it all the time.
* I liked that and I may enjoy it again sometime.
* It was okay but I don't have big feelings about it either way.

* I didn't like it because I may have done it wrong.
* I didn't like it and I never want to do that again.

And that's it. If you don't like something, you really don't ever need to do it again. Except go to work, unfortunately. That's one of those things that, even if we don't like it, we can't really opt out of. Damn capitalism.

We are of the opinion that, unless you absolutely hated your experience of something to the point of it traumatizing you, almost everything is worth trying twice. Trying again is a proven scientific way to determine if you want to nope out forever or if it's suddenly now your favorite thing. Now, it's important to note that, should you absolutely hate something and find yourself no longer even remotely intrigued by it, this advice needn't be followed. But if you tried it and feel like it just didn't jibe, or your partner moved weird, or you couldn't get in a good position, you may want to give it another go.

Is Pegging a Kink?

Yes and no.

Helpful, right? While the more mainstream public might label pegging as a kink, or kinky, those in the BDSM community may well scoff and suggest that pegging is just sex with extra steps. The acronym BDSM stands for a lot of things, but mostly refers to bondage, discipline, sadomasochism, masochism, Dom, sub, slave, and/or Master. The term BDSM has become shorthand for the umbrella that covers most kinks, fetishes, or sexually alternative lifestyles.

One of the reasons pegging is so often considered part of BDSM is the perceived Dominant/submissive nature of the act. This ties in with the role reversal we mentioned earlier, but it goes deeper than that. To suggest that one must be dominant or in the dominant role in order to be the pegger, and one must be submissive to be the peggee, really begs us to look at the generalized roles of men and women in sexuality.

If, as a vagina-haver, you only ever receive penetration, does this automatically make you submissive? As a penis-haver doing the penetration, are you the dominant? Sex itself isn't about dominance and submission, as those are only values we imbue into it. Acknowledging that sometimes the woman being fucked is definitely the dominant, and the man fucking is definitely being submissive recognizes that pegging is the same way.

While elements of kink and BDSM can absolutely be applied to pegging, the way they can be applied to any other type of sex, inherently, by itself, pegging is not BDSM. It's up to you whether you want to consider it kinky. After all, it wasn't that long ago that having sex with the lights on may have also been called kinky.

The Prostate Orgasm

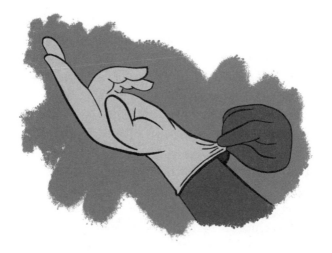

Scientists won't even agree that the G-spot is a thing, so they aren't about to start talking about prostate orgasms. Luckily, we're not scientists, nor do we get our funding restricted when Mothers Against Fun come screaming. So, that's not what this chapter is about, but we feel compelled to come down hard on the side of *The G-Spot is Real*. But truly, we shouldn't have to do that.

The prostate orgasm is real, too. We've seen it. Cooper has had them (stay tuned for a story about that). So, don't let anybody try to convince you otherwise. These are the same folks who try to downplay squirting orgasms in women.

For most men, orgasms are one and done. You squirt and the turtle goes back into his shell for a long nap. It feels great, of course, but there's actually very little happening in the moment between buildup and afterglow. It's a lot like a sneeze, something huge and involuntary that has the potential to make a mess.

Sure, there are some penis-havers lucky enough to be able to come again and again and again, until there's nothing left and it's like someone dropped a bag of flour in there. They may or may not need the refractory period to soften and then grow hard again. These are lucky men. And they're rare.

Still others are unable to orgasm at all, or only orgasm in very specific ways. Or ejaculation itself is off the menu.

Well, as the man says, what if we could show you an even better way?

Now, we don't actually believe prostate orgasms are *better* than penile/ejaculatory orgasms, because what's really being ranked in that comparison are orgasms and orgasms. However, for most, they are very different.

While the ejaculation orgasm has been compared to a sneeze (you saw, we compared it!), most prostate orgasms are like waves lapping on a beautiful island shore.

To take a side jaunt here, let's talk about the G-spot and squirting orgasms. Not all women can have them (and not all who have them are women) but those who can squirt will often tell you how different they are from clitoral orgasms. When they describe these "different" orgasms, they too will liken them to waves.

The wave orgasm begins much the same way that an ejaculatory orgasm does. You know that point in a blowjob when you might tap your partner and say "I'm close" so she doesn't get a sudden cum-load unexpectedly? Well, that's the rising wave. The big difference here with the prostate orgasm over the penile is that when that wave crests, usually you're not spurting cum.

This means a sensation that builds and builds and builds and a climax that arrives and sticks around. Because it takes time for that cresting wave to crash upon the shore and roll back. And like a rolling wave, it's not finished, it just reaches its ebb and comes rolling back up. Which, as you may have guessed, means multiple orgasms. No refractory period.

Or maybe just one massive orgasm. The sea isn't defined by the number of waves, after all.

Regardless of whether semantically it's coming once, or twice, or infinity times, it's no longer the sneeze-like shot and recuperating time. The waves keep rising and breaking and rolling back until they're done.

What does it feel like if not a sneeze?

Intensity itself. As we mentioned, it's like that "I'm close" build, so just picture following that through beyond the point where ejaculation would happen, that intensity increasing and increasing until it breaks and rolls back, giving you a moment to collect yourself and breathe before the wave crashes back in.

For Cooper, these waves are accompanied by intense shaking that ebbs and flows at the same time. The sensation is like that great feeling after a stretch, where it's really intense for a moment and then becomes a calming good feeling. An *ahhhhhhhh*.

We've had the good fortune of speaking with many people about many types of orgasms, across body types, across gender expressions, and nearly every person we've spoken to who has these types of secondary orgasms (not a hierarchy, there's just a notable division at first between clit/penis orgasms and G-spot/prostate orgasms) does one other interesting thing.

At first, prostate orgasms (and G-spot ones, and gushing) are rare, elusive. You may not know if you even had one if you did. It may feel like other types, it may feel like nothing you've ever felt before, but once your body locks in on that, things begin to change.

So, for a time you may only be able to have the prostate orgasm, the wave orgasm, the rolling orgasm through very specific touch in very specific instances. But then suddenly you're feeling the wave during blowjobs or handjobs, during penetrative sex. Sometimes the new pathways are so strong you can call the wave from the slightest touch.

Sometimes it's too much. But not often.

Cooper has been nagging to tell the tale of his first prostate orgasm, so we'll let him do that. It wasn't pegging, but, as you can imagine, it changed him.

It Won't Stop: The Epic Prostate Orgasm

An excerpt from My Life on the Swingset: Adventures in Swinging & Polyamory by Cooper S. Beckett

I've been chasing the prostate orgasm for months, perhaps years now, the way many women chase that elusive first G-spot orgasm. While some assholes may still question the existence of a G-spot, there's no doubt that the prostate exists. The question is, rather: can it produce pleasure on its own?

I'd heard tell around the campfire, my friends, about the orgasm without ejaculation, conjured from prostate stimulation. I was told it could be long, multiple, and unlike anything I'd ever experienced (namely short and single). After all, our bodies are designed so once the cum shoots out, the shop gets closed up, the lights get turned off, and our balls say, "you don't have to go home, but you can't stay here."

I think I'd once come close with a very special friend who was intent on focusing on me instead of her. She had me feeling all sorts of unique and new sensations before putting her mouth on me to finish the job. That orgasm had an ejaculation, indeed, but the erection didn't immediately subside. It looked like someone forgot to turn off the lights. The factory was still running.

This fascinated me because that never happens. I'm one of those people who, once I come, the chemicals produced change my point of view so dramatically that I feel like I never need to have sex again. Been there, done that, bought the t-shirt.

I'd never known anyone who'd actually managed a prostate orgasm. Compared to it, the G-spot orgasm may be elusive, but was fairly common among the open women in my social circle. Not only that, but most of them also seemed not to care that it might be a thing.

But I cared. I cared big-time.

Much of my definition of sex has been caught up in that white, jizzy final expulsion. Since I know myself, and that I have that "closed for business entirely" sensibility after an orgasm, I tend to put my partner's pleasure first. Once she has had an orgasm, or many, only then do I allow myself to head in that direction. The idea of an orgasm that wouldn't end things for me is tremendously appealing.

The problems with chasing such an orgasm are myriad. It's a sensitive area indeed. The first prostate orgasm, much like a first G-spot orgasm, requires a lot of time, concentration, and effort to bring forth.

If they exist at all, that is. Tristan Taormino has assured me that they do, as not only has she seen one, but she's conjured one. Of course, if Tristan laid those beautiful hands on me, in me…I got lost in thought.

Where was I?

All this talk about the possibility that they don't exist is silly, though, isn't it? Especially now that I've had one.

Oh, yes.

Yesterday, on a bed near the rooftop hot tub at Desire Resort and Spa in sunny Cancún, as I enjoyed demonstrating the nJoy Eleven on a very willing friend, I asked if someone might insert my favorite butt plug, handmade by the incredibly talented Boris.

A volunteer came forward, a beautiful woman with whom I'd shared a lot of eye contact and some kisses at our speed dating event. I was assured she was a professional (though I wasn't certain what that meant at the time) and that I shouldn't worry. I wasn't worried to begin with, but I thanked her for volunteering, for her enthusiasm, and returned my attention to the Eleven and my lovely playmate.

My volunteer didn't step back after insertion. She continued to manipulate, pressing the plug, moving it in and out, circling it. Before long I was distracted. Then I could no longer continue with the Eleven. Thankfully my playmate had brought out her LELO Siri and whispered that she might have had enough of the massive Eleven. I continued to kneel above her as she played with herself, responding compersively to my spasms that were growing more frequent from the anal stimulation.

Before long I couldn't support myself on my hands and knees. My lovely playmate below suggested that I lie next to her and took my hand. My volunteer asked if I was doing alright, if it was too much, touching my arm and thigh as she asked. Tremendously comforting. "I'm very comfortable saying 'Ouch, ouch, that hurts!'" I told her.

"Promise?"

I promised.

She became more aggressive, moving her whole body in rhythm, gripping my thigh and my arm at times, putting her hand on my chest to gain leverage, to hold me down, to push the energy right into me.

Somewhere in there, it started.

I've always achieved small spasms during prostate play, the kind of spasms you hit as your cock is being played with, those early signposts that you're going in the right direction. With prostate stimulation, these moments were usually brief but very pleasurable. But on that bed, with this expert, I found these spasms elongating and coming closer together, becoming tremors and full-body shaking. Bigger and bigger, closer and closer, until the gap between them disappeared.

Here's where it all gets fuzzy and dreamlike. Once the gap vanished it was like a wave rushing toward shore that wasn't breaking, and the shore just moved back at the same speed as the wave. On and on the shakiness rolled, spasming, rocking my body. I couldn't breathe. I couldn't think.

"Shh, don't clench," she whispered to me, running her fingers along my very tense legs. My hands were indeed clenched into tight fists. I opened them and put my head back down.

"Just breathe."

This continued for the better part of an hour. At least I think so. I honestly have no idea because time had fractured and lost meaning. I may have been orgasming for decades or only a minute. I've since been assured it was almost fifty minutes from the beginning of the "clearly orgasmic" portion of my time on that bed to the end.

When I threw the flag down and tapped out.

I thanked her; words unable to accurately reflect my gratitude. She assured me that I had indeed progressed through many and varied orgasms if my face and body were any indication. As I lay there, basking for a while, a curious thing happened. An aftershock tremor hit, causing me to curl up my knees to my chest—an ecstatic moment of orgasmic delight.

This by itself was surprising enough, but these tremors continued during the walk back to my room, during the shower before dinner, while getting food from the buffet (I had to ask a friend to get me a deviled egg because I couldn't hold the tongs steady), and through on to dessert. Only after sitting at dinner for an hour or so did the tremors finally begin to subside.

A nearly endless orgasm with the vast capacity for more. Without the standard feelings of "Okay, I'm done." A whole new world. How thrilling that is. After all, I'm no longer chasing the possibly mythical prostate orgasm.

Now I'm just chasing the very real next prostate orgasm.

O, happy day!

Read more essays by Cooper in *My Life on the Swingset: Adventures in Swinging & Polyamory.*

Other Thoughts on Prostate Orgasms

It is worth noting that because, like the G-spot and its accompanying orgasms, prostate orgasms aren't really "recognized by society," you won't be able to find a single definitive source on what a prostate orgasm is or feels like. As much as your authors may enjoy being called a definitive source, we're not; we're only speaking from our experience. Your prostate orgasm may be the aforementioned wave, yours may be intensity in your stomach, yours may even include ejaculation.

With that in mind, we encourage you to have a paradigm shift. Sounds big, doesn't it? Well, that's because it kind of is.

A paradigm shift is a monumental shift in the way of thinking. The most profound example was way back when people went from thinking of the Earth as the center of the solar system to the sun being the center.

What does this have to do with pegging?

Well, it's not pegging directly—we'd like you to have a paradigm shift in how you think about sex in general. It's tempting to follow the societal conceit that sex is "penis in vagina penetration." Those who have this conceit will often begrudgingly allow it to accommodate "penis in anus penetration." Honestly, it was not that long ago when your authors thought this too, so don't feel bad if that's what you think or have thought.

Honestly, much of society looks at it that way, and if not specifying the direct ingredients of the penetration, they definitely see sex as something that must involve penetration. By this definition, pegging does in fact equal sex, so where's the paradigm shift?

We want you to expand the definition of sex by taking out the need for penetration. Because sex isn't penetration. Sex is penetration and oral sex and foreplay and rubbing each other and handjobs and every sexual thing. Sex has never been exclusively penetration, except to people who don't much care about their partners' orgasms.

Once we expand our notions of sex to include all of those things, and include them whether or not orgasms are had, it can be especially emotionally freeing. Definitely for those who've ever felt less-than if they don't have orgasms or they cannot stay hard to penetrate.

Now that we've separated and expanded the word sex, let's look conceptually at "the orgasm."

First off, orgasms are awesome—we can all agree on that. And they can range in awesomeness from the grateful release of a sneeze to a seemingly endless series of waves lapping on the shore. They can be plentiful for some, easy to achieve, even early, or they can be ever elusive and difficult to track down. The variance of how, when, and why we orgasm could be the subject of its own book.

But beyond that, the difference between internal orgasms and ejaculatory orgasms can be very different. Partly this is down to function. As awesome as ejaculating from a penis is (and, it is), it serves a very important biological function, and that is the perpetuation of the human race. (No pressure.) Because deep down we're all animals, and this biological imperative is there, it's designed very specifically to fire off the baby juice and then shut down the system so Grog can focus on the all-important hunting and gathering. This is why almost immediately after an ejaculatory orgasm, the penises of most men return to their flaccid state.

It may seem negative to note that the female orgasm doesn't serve an evolutionary function, but in truth it's rather lucky. Because that orgasm literally only exists for pleasure. So, while the male ejaculatory orgasm is designed as a one-and-done-er that can possibly reload with some refractory time, the internal orgasm can roll on and on and on, since that one comes down to pleasurable muscle spasms.

When people first decide to try pegging, they may watch a lot of pegging porn, which often shows rock-hard men being fucked in the ass and jizzing all over the place. The reality is, because of the way the prostate and penis are wired separately, ejaculation rarely accompanies prostate orgasms at the beginning.

To vagina-havers who began to have squirting orgasms, though, this next part may seem familiar.

Once a prostate orgasm is achieved, it's almost as though an entirely new set of neurons have lit up across the sexiest parts of your brain. And the more they light up, the more they send their sexy tendrils out to attach to other things. Therefore, while early prostate play may involve simple orgasms or none at all, soon those tendrils reach the areas of the brain responsible for ejaculation and penile play.

Cooper can attest, once the prostate orgasm switch was flipped, the waves of intense prostate orgasm began to show up without any prostate stimulation at all.

All this talk of orgasms, though, neglects to mention the most important thing. In the grand scheme of sexual exploration, orgasms are *not* as important as we've been led to believe. We think they are, of course, mostly because orgasms are generally the "end" of sex when we see it in movies, TV, and porn. (Talking male ejaculatory orgasms here, because society has placed an absurd level of import on them.) This pedestal placement can lead to us thinking we've somehow failed if we cannot come.

And bottom line, folks. In all of our lives, there will be dry spells. Cum droughts, if you will.

So, because prostate orgasms are often brand-new for those first experiencing pegging, we advise you to try to take the focus off the orgasm. It may not happen right away, or at all, and if your entire focus is on getting there, you may not pay attention to all the amazing things that are happening in your body on that road.

Awesome sex, like life, is about the journey.

The Leaking Prostate

It's worth mentioning here that, while ejaculatory orgasms won't always happen with prostate play and pegging, the prostate is where the stuff that makes ejaculation possible comes from. In the simplest terms, the prostate provides the ships for the sperms to make their (e)missions.

Anyway, the prostate produces (surprise, surprise) prostatic fluid, and when you squeeze the prostate, or press against it, or massage it, this fluid can be squeezed out. You've seen it before—it's usually called pre-cum. That clear sticky bit that shows up when you're having a good time, just early enough to get on your pants.

So, prostate play, especially extended play like pegging, will probably squeeze out enough prostatic fluid to get drippy. If you're on your knees while the pegging is going down, you should probably put a towel below you because otherwise it's getting on the sheets.

More advanced prostate players will sometimes "milk the prostate" in order to squeeze out a significant amount of this prostatic fluid. Coincidentally, sometimes doctors will do this, too, as it can be a treatment for prostate issues. The pleasure derived from the two variants of this act can and should be different.

But What About...?

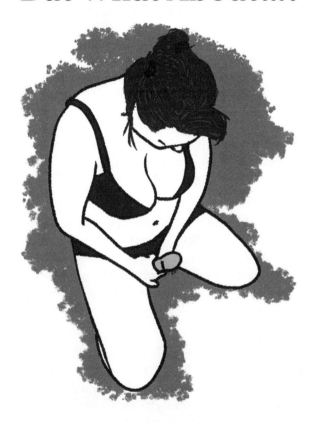

If you're anything like us, you probably get in your head a bit when considering things, especially new and potentially scary (sounding) sex. Because we understand this thoroughly, we're going to do our best to address the...stuff...that can get in the way of you enjoying your pegging experience, from the social, to the emotional, to the physical.

Social Stigma

As we have said, no sexual act can change your sexual orientation or identity. There's no light switch in your butt that reads "gay" on top and "hetero" on the bottom that could be flipped simply by stimulating some awesome nerve endings in your rectum.

At its core, pegging is sex, no matter how big and scary it can seem to those new to the act. It's sticking something in a bodily orifice with the goal of bringing about pleasure. That's sex, folks, plain and simple. And at its most basic level, sex between a man and a woman is now and will always be heterosexual sex. But let's not make it sound *too* boring now.

For as heterocentric an act as pegging technically is, it brings with it a lot of social stigma. As educators, the most common questions we get often begin with "How do I convince my partner to..." and then the person asking will usually drop to a whisper when they put a name to the act. Most of the time, our answer is the same: "You could, y'know, ask them..." But the phrasing and desire of the question speaks to the big bad that surrounds sex in our culture.

Shame.

Why wouldn't we just tell our partners anything and everything we're interested in trying? Especially in a long-term relationship, we should be over the shyness of asking for what we want, shouldn't we?

In an ideal world, yes, we should. But we live in this one, where we've been shamed for our sexual interests since the beginning, and then as we grow up are told there's "normal sex" (which we're still getting shamed for) and "deviant sex" (for which übershame is reserved). So, we're afraid of the same thing we've always been afraid of. Being laughed at, having our partner go "eew, pervert!" Cooper's personal fear is always being knocked down, laughed at, kicked in the balls, and left.

We won't tell you it's unheard of for a partner to be surprised, even shocked, by a sexual desire. It could happen. It's why we advocate communicating early, often, and constantly thereafter. Otherwise going from a fairly vanilla missionary-only-on-weekends sex life to "tie me up and fuck my ass" may very well cause some surprise and consternation.

That said, communicating your desires to a partner is incredibly important in virtually all aspects of a relationship. You probably already do a lot of it every day. Want to get spanked? Want to have kids one day? Want to be celibate for a period of time? All of these kinds of desires are important to discuss with a partner, not because your partner can cast the deciding vote in what you get to do with your body, but they do have control in what they do with *their* body, and ultimately get to decide whether or not to stay in a relationship if they can't meet your needs, or you can't meet theirs.

Asking about your wants and desires can be compared to the Schrödinger's cat experiment.

The gist of Schrödinger's cat is that there's a cat inside a closed box with poisoned food. With the box closed, we don't know if the cat has eaten the food, so we don't know if it is alive or dead. We know it's a depressing concept, but the experiment is meant to demonstrate a dual state that can only be understood by observing it.

In other words, *you have to open the box*.

Because in practice, it's not actually a dual state, but three possibilities. One, you open the box and the cat's alive, so you get to play with the cat. Yay! Two, you open the box and the cat's dead, so you don't get to play with the cat. Sad. Three, you don't open the box. You don't get to play with the cat. This one's on you.

So, literally the only way to get the happy ending is to open the box. And the sad result when you open the box is the same as if you didn't open it at all. Doing nothing is the same as getting a negative result.

Go with us here—let's apply this to specifically asking your partner to peg you.

You ask, they say yes, you get pegged.

You ask, they say no, you don't get pegged.

You don't ask, you don't get pegged.

This is something that we all objectively know, even if we manage to talk ourselves out of it. Nothing ventured, nothing gained. It isn't just an adage, it's the fucking truth. The only way we get to do cool things is by deciding to explore. And if you're sitting around waiting for your partner to come to you and ask you to do the exact thing you've been jacking off over for years...well, it could happen, but we don't like your odds.

This isn't to say that there isn't risk in sharing these things with a partner. Some people have been long taught that anything involving the butt is disgusting, or gay, or sinful. Some may have strong feelings about the act. In extreme cases, some may even consider the idea a RELE (Relationship Extinction-Level Event). So, we won't sugarcoat it and promise that all will come up roses.

What we will do is gently suggest that having open and honest communication about urges and desires is one of the most valuable things you can do in a relationship. Fantasy life can sometimes be a minefield, because we don't know what may trigger others. But we stand by the principle that you should strive toward open and honest communication, because once you reach it, everything looks brighter.

This isn't the book for it, but it's worth taking a moment to recognize that sometimes people simply aren't sexually compatible. What you do with that information is up to each individual relationship as a whole and each person in it. For some, this means exploration together to see if you can find compatibility. For some, it means breaking up to find sexual compatibility with another person. For others, it means opening up your relationship so you can find the sex you desire with another person while keeping your relationship together for the value it has. Whatever your course, all that matters is what the people within the relationship think. Fuck the world.

We know that previous paragraph got all "real" and stuff. It's a hard point, but it's true. The first question most people ask about pegging, even in relationships where communication is solid, is "How do I convince my partner/girlfriend/boyfriend...?" The idea of convincing immediately assumes that the answer is going to be a no, and that you'll have to figure out a way around that no. But we advise you to work your way past that thought. Because you're not trying to convince or coerce or cajole or any other C-word like that. You're expressing a desire that you have and asking if your partner shares it or is curious about that.

The next common question that shares the same origins in shame is "How do I tell my partner that I'm into..."

So, how do you tell your partner you're into being pegged, when society tells you as a man you're supposed to be on top, to be dominant, to be the fucker, not the fuckee? A willingness to be vulnerable is essential here. To come right out and say, "So, I'm kinda interested in this thing..." But sometimes even that is hard. So, we're gonna give you a shortcut.

Find out which streaming service near you has the Comedy Central show *Broad City* on it. Sit down with your partner and cue up Season Two, Episode Four, "Knockoffs," also known as "The Pegging Episode." In this episode, Abbi (Abbi Jacobson) is given the opportunity to peg the new man in her life. The entire episode is full of discussion on the act, as well as people curiously asking questions about it. It includes a delightful moment when national treasure Bob Balaban wonders if he would like it.

So, you've watched this episode, and laughed, and learned, and loved. Now, really, all it takes is a simple question: "What do you think of that?" (More examples, both good and bad, of pegging in popular media are coming for you in the next section!)

Conversations aren't nearly as difficult as beginning them might suggest. And you may not, of course, need to watch Abbi's pegging journey to start this conversation with your partner (though it's still hilarious and worth watching). Having compassion for your partner's interests, even if the initial idea may squick you, is essential to a happy and healthy sexual relationship.

What if they say no?

They might. For myriad reasons. And if they say they're not interested, you need to respect that. As much as we proselytize to "Never yuck anyone else's yum," you also shouldn't make a habit of trying to change someone's yuck into a yum. If someone is uncomfortable with the idea of anal sex now, it doesn't necessarily mean they will be forever, but it does mean that they are not into it right now, and you need to be okay with that. Either way, you're planting a seed in their brain that may grow into something later. It might become a new porn search term. It might spark something in them they didn't realize they had an interest in. It might turn into a turn-on and become a yum one day. Be patient with a lover when exploring the unknown, because someday they're likely going to ask you to explore something you're nervous about.

One caveat we'd like to address if you're an unpartnered man reading this. Your question may be, "How exactly do I find someone to peg me?"

Well, to that we want to say, "Please don't." Not that you shouldn't explore pegging by any means— you should—but please don't try to find a new partner whose sole purpose in your life is simply to peg you.

If you're on dating sites, or, worse yet, social networking sites, and you make a habit of messaging women asking them if they'd be up for pegging you, you will be branded a Grade-A creep. Lyndzi regularly has to deal with such things due to having pegging listed as an interest on some dating sites and the fact that we teach a class on the topic. She's had *many* of these types of messages: "Do you do home demonstrations?" "Can I be the bottom in your class?" (It's not that kind of class.) "My ass is ready. What do I have to do to get you to experiment on me?" These dudes will often ask these questions as their *very first* message. Cue the eye roll and grimace.

This isn't to say there's anything wrong with looking to date someone or connect with someone who might be interested in pegging you. We're just saying that it absolutely should not be your number-one focus. As with anything else you look for in a partner or playmate, it should be a part of a vast tapestry of overlapping interests. Just as you don't immediately whip your penis out when saying hello on a first date (or at least you absolutely SHOULD NOT do this), you should not whip out your sexual kinks immediately. They should be approached when the subject moves to the type of sex you both might be interested in having.

Slightly different rules apply on sexually focused dating/networking sites, like Fetlife or any of the various hookup apps. Still, we advise treating pegging like dick pics. Sometimes they're appropriate, but only when the conversational desire is there. Usually, they're as unwelcome as the big Dick, Nixon, himself in the conversation.

If all of this seems exhausting and you are desperate to get right to the pegging, there is another option, of course. There are oodles of skilled sex workers out there, and many do specialize in pegging as one of their primary offerings. There is absolutely nothing wrong with going in this direction, and we fully support those who are sex workers, and those who pay sex workers handsomely (and treat them wonderfully) for their sexual prowesses.

Butt Stuff Experiences & Interests

You and your partner/playmate should each fill
this out separately and compare notes afterward.

Receiving			Giving			
Done It	Into It	No Thanks	Done It	Into It	No Thanks	
☐	☐	☐	☐	☐	☐	Fingering around the outside
☐	☐	☐	☐	☐	☐	Toying around the outside
☐	☐	☐	☐	☐	☐	Licking around the outside
☐	☐	☐	☐	☐	☐	Finger insertion
☐	☐	☐	☐	☐	☐	Tongue insertion
☐	☐	☐	☐	☐	☐	Butt plug use
☐	☐	☐	☐	☐	☐	Long-term butt plug use (60 min+)
☐	☐	☐	☐	☐	☐	Anal beads use
☐	☐	☐	☐	☐	☐	Dildo use/thrusting
☐	☐	☐	☐	☐	☐	Pegging
☐	☐	☐	☐	☐	☐	Anal fisting

Media Representations of Pegging

In the course of mainstream cinematic history, pegging and/or anal sex has been depicted only a handful of times. Positively? Not as much as we would hope. We have discovered a couple of portrayals of pegging in particular, which we go into in this section, but, honestly, almost all left something to be desired. Aside from *Broad City*, even the most positive of these depictions are used, sadly enough, as the *butt* of a joke (ugh, what a horrible dad joke), and the worst are just straight-up sexual assault. It's pretty fucked-up, but we think it's important to see the state of play on the act, as the general tone of the media reflects societal acceptance of pegging. As more people accept, more people explore, more people peg, stigma will gradually fade away, and more shows will be like *Broad City*, showing pegging to be awesome!

Broad City (Season 2, Episode 4, "Knockoffs," 2015)
This is probably our favorite and one of the most positive depictions of pegging. The act is brought up due to a miscommunication, but the protagonist Abbi rolls with it after consulting her very excited, pegging-enthused friend Ilana. The pegging is consensual and both parties seem genuinely excited and a little nervous. Ilana is *so* excited about Abbi getting the opportunity to peg that she has to take a moment to twerk upside down in celebration. The show is

a comedy, but it never takes a shot at shaming the male character who wants to be pegged. The comedy is centered more on Abbi's hesitation and Ilana's pure delight at the prospect that her bestie is going to pop her pegging cherry.

Deadpool (2016)

Though this scene is only a few seconds long, it definitely leaves a lasting impression. The act seems to be consensual, but it's also used as a joke within a holiday montage, this being how the main character and his girlfriend celebrate National Women's Day. Deadpool is on all fours, his partner Vanessa kneeling behind him in a harness. It's alluded to that she penetrates him, he looks tense, and he whispers "No" to himself a couple times. It's not shown whether or not his partner stops because the scene ends there, but in the sequel Deadpool jokes that he's going to get the strap-on so they can try to make a baby. Vanessa replies, "I don't think that's how it works, but we can try," hinting that Deadpool enjoys pegging now. Either way, seeing Vanessa in a harness is a sight that stops both of our bisexual hearts, so there's at least that.

Weeds (Season 2, Episode 6, "Crush Girl Love Panic," 2006)
On the scale of positive to negative depictions, this one falls into the negative realm. The male character is hesitant at best when his very attractive date whips

out a huge black dildo and straps it on, clearly stating his unease and non-consent. Pegging at that point would be at best coercive, at worst literal assault. The woman says, "It will fit," mockingly, when the man seems concerned about her *gigantic* dildo, before she rips off his boxers. There's absolutely no negotiation and the scene is played off as a joke.

Shameless (Season 1, Episode 2, "Frank the Plank," 2011) This one is not really pegging, just anal penetration with a dildo, but we thought it was worth mentioning because it is *so* bad. It's not only non-consensual—the character is cuffed to the bed and not given a choice—but a dildo is used on him while he literally screams "Stop" (which he and his partner agreed would be their safeword). In the next scene, he's shown limping bowlegged down the stairs, apparently for laughs, then his partner makes him a nice dinner and gives him a pillow to sit on, which he does, as if everything is hunky-dory. Wow, this depiction sucks a lot! Calling it non-consensual is being delicate, because it's honestly depicting rape. Full stop. 0/10 do not recommend.

The Sopranos (Season 4, Episode 3, "Christopher," 2002) This scene is quick but consensual, with the act being interrupted by a phone call. The male character, Ralph, puts down a vial that we assume to be poppers, before taking the call. This character is depicted as kinky and called a sexual deviant by other characters. This definitely aligns with the show's views of what a man's role is in sex, as earlier in the series there is a lot of hubbub about going down on women being not so manly. Definitely intended to make the audience judge both the kink and the pegging.

Horrible Bosses 2 (2014)

This two-second scene depicts a woman pegging a man caught on a security camera. It's likely consensual, and the man seems very happy afterward, but it is overall played off as a joke, with borderline homophobic tones.

Zack and Miri Make a Porno (2008)

This pegging scene is overall positive. It's a quick shot of two porn stars consensually engaging in pegging for a porn film. The two are friendly with one another and seem to have a great time. The movie kind of codes that male character as gay but never says so outright. This gave us icky feelings because it's as if the movie is saying that being penetrated anally is something only gay guys do, since none of the coded-straight characters get pegged. That said, it is a Kevin Smith movie, so there probably wasn't a whole lot of deep thought going on.

There are a few more depictions of pegging on film and screen, and there will hopefully be many more to come, but these are the top hits for a taste of what Hollywood has to offer so far. Which is, sadly, pretty pathetic. Let's hope that the future brings mainstream representations of pegging as the fun and awesome act that it is, and not just a joke.

Internalized Misogyny and Fragile Masculinity

There are many toxic things in our world and in our brains that steal joy. Misogyny and ego are some of the worst offenders of this joy-thievery. Though misogyny is often thought of as a problem of men's attitudes and behaviors toward women, there's also the internalized form that sprouts up in women, which can be just as toxic. Internalized misogyny is the sexist and misogynistic thoughts held by women about themselves or about other women. These hard-held beliefs can lead to behaviors that are shitty to both the person holding them and to other women. General misogyny is often created and reinforced by society's attitude. It's used to further oppress women and keep them "in their place" but can, and often does, affect men too. Misogyny has been a tool to prevent equality for...well, ever. The patriarchal brainwashing of society runs deep and can be hard to undo, even for the people who are being actively oppressed.

Fragile masculinity, on the other hand, feels like the other side of this toxic, rotten coin. It's the anxiety of men feeling as though they can never be "man" enough, as set by our patriarchal standards for masculinity. Don't eat rare steak while riding a horse bareback with your ax and gun at the ready? Then how can you even call yourself a man? It's horseshit, but it's what is crammed into the brains of boys from early on.

The depictions of "masculine" men do the same kind of damage to men's self-esteem as Photoshopped, wafer-thin Victoria's Secret models do to young girls' body image. Both make folks feel lesser and like they will never be the "perfect" version of man or woman that society is screaming that they must be. These role models can lead to eating disorders, a lack of body acceptance, anxiety, and/or depression, and in men, the concept of being "strong" can also lead to threatening behaviors, with the idea that strength equals violence.

When we spoke with Andre Shakti, she addressed both of these phenomena. "Unfortunately, in our society in the year 2022," Shakti said, "we still have a really unhealthy perception of masculinity and what it means to be, 'masculine versus non-masculine.'...And we tell them exactly what it means to be a masculine man, whether it's overtly or whether it's more so like mainstream media, school, friends, family structures, etc. We reward certain kinds of behavior and deem [them] more masculine. So that young men will seek out those behaviors and experiences, and something that is afforded to young men from a very early age, again subtly and/or overtly, is that your ass is an exit-only location. That if you seek to derive any pleasure from anal stimulation of any kind, that makes you homosexual."

As we have discussed, no amount of butt play *makes* a person gay, but the fragility around being manly still exists, and the idea of being penetrated is culturally considered the least manly thing a man can do, because that's the "woman's job." Men are the fuckers, they fuck, and women are the fucked.

"Out of an abundance of caution and fear, and anxiety and reticence about how they might be read, in particular by other men, if they dare to explore that part of their body," Shakti went on, "many young men close themselves off to anal pleasure, because again, of this idea that A) it must be somehow inherently connected to a desire for sexual stimulation from other men, and B) someone will find out and they will then be deemed less masculine and then lose respect, and potentially opportunities, especially again in the eyes of the close men in their life. So, we really do a number on guys."

When it comes to women's ideas of masculinity and femininity, they are not free of the cultural bullshit that men are subjected to, and some react pretty negatively. Shakti continued, "It really pains me to see the way in which so many women have internalized misogyny and play out that misogyny in their everyday lives, and I fucking see it played out in their reactions and responses to their male partners seeking anal pleasure. It is such a mind-fucky devastating thing to hear about and watch."

"You know, when I do get my clients," Shakti said about her job as a sex worker, "when guys do hit me up for pegging solo, inevitably, at some point during our first session, I always ask them, 'So, just out of curiosity, are you involved with anybody? Do you have a girlfriend? Do you have a wife?' And if they respond positively, I ask. 'Well, have you tried talking to her about it?' Which is probably bad for my business, right? But I'm an educator at heart. And I know that so many men are coming to me not because they don't want to, but kind of as a second resort, or last resort, because their own partners refuse to fulfill and/or heavily shame and stigmatize them for wanting to fulfill certain desires."

Lyndzi here: Something I see regularly at the sex-toy store I work at is folks joking around the anal toy section. Whether they're awkward and it gives them the giggles (hey, butts are funny, I'll give them that) or they're nervous because it's actually something they're into but don't want anyone else to know, the natural way to deal with that nervousness is to joke about it. On the more insidious side of these jokes are the women who say things along the lines of, "If you let your man do that, you might as well be a dude." Or, "If my guy wanted that, I'd tell him to get his ass out of bed and make *me* a sandwich." The sexism so often pointed at them for being the "weaker sex" gets viciously twisted and turned around.

I get really sad when I hear these kinds of comments. I wonder how insecure these ladies are in their relationships to think that any kind of consensual act with their partner, an act meant to give pleasure, would make said partner completely change their life and up and leave them for someone of the same sex. I think about how horrible the men in the rest of the store must feel, having to overhear women talk about them in such a way. I know how that feels, after all—it's how a lot of men talk about women.

At its core, internalized misogyny is a way for women to truly hate themselves. They compare men who get penetrated to women, as if that's the worst thing someone can be. They worry that a man wanting anal play means he actually wants to be with men, because who wouldn't prefer men to women (women being the lowly beings that they are)? Ultimately, these ideas are saying that being like a woman in any way is repulsive and wrong.

How do we combat this prevailing idea that "woman" means flawed, lesser, or bad? How do we as a society change the minds of men *and* women to believe that being feminine is just as worthy as being masculine? That being a strong man doesn't mean being violent, but that it means being brave, vulnerable, and secure in one's own masculinity *as well as* one's own femininity. That being feminine doesn't mean being weak, but that it means being powerful and resilient. Not fragile like a flower, Frida Kahlo would say, but fragile like a bomb.

This revolutionary way of thinking can start in the bedroom. It starts with all of us looking into our biases, questioning them, and, if need be, changing them. What beliefs do you hold about masculinity and femininity? Are any of them based on toxic stereotypes? Think about how you can personally reframe these ideas. We change the world by changing one mind at a time.

The Anal Shame Effect

Sometimes in life we encounter a coincidence, something that has happened to more than just us, and it's tempting to then apply that phenomenon to the whole world, because we crave shared experiences.

But if that phenomenon keeps coming up with so many people that we talk to, it's gotta be a *thing*, right?

With that dubious lead-in, we'd like to talk about the feelings of shame that can accompany pegging and anal play. As we discuss the social stigma that surrounds the act, we must also discuss the internal shame that can accompany it. There are many reasons that we might have internalized shame, and that in itself is nothing of which to be ashamed.

That said, many men will talk about odd feelings of shame that accompany anal play and settle upon them either during or just after the act. This feeling is similar to the self-loathing that can arise post-masturbation orgasm in some who grew up believing that what they're doing is something they should feel bad about.

So many of us grew up with strong shame and prejudice against sex in general, both created by and compounded by a societal view that's mainly shaped by religious or other so-called "moral" teachings. Most of these worldviews perceive sex as, if not simply for procreation, then, well, you shouldn't be having too much fun with it. And God forbid if you get *creative!*

But even as many move beyond and out of that mindset, the deep inner core remains. That shame can be triggered intensely because of the simple intensity of the act of pegging. It's something that requires more bodily commitment, and activates more nerves than PIV sex, so it's firing up a lot more locations in your brain, and some of them may still be wired into that shame box.

The only thing for us to do is, first, realize we shouldn't be ashamed of feeling shame. This doesn't mean we're actually judging ourselves or our partners. It just means we have a bit of a blockage to work through. Working through it can include things as simple as seeing how much fun you or your partner have and realizing that it's not affecting anybody but yourselves. Why should we be ashamed of things that hurt literally no one?

Physical Limitations

As with most other sex acts, pegging may be more difficult for people with physical limitations. Limited mobility or inability to thrust can lead you to believe pegging may not be for you. In our later section on positioning, we make note of issues this may cause. But pegging need not be beyond your grasp. Adapting positioning, changing who is responsible for the thrusting (back-it-up can be just as effective as pushing it forward!) can be solutions. But as with any other sex act, limited mobility or other physical limitations should not make you feel excluded from the act, and with patient discussions and planning (perhaps a whiteboard), you'll be able to find your specific version of pegging that works for your bodies.

Conversation Stimulation

For this exercise, we'll ask you to fill this out separately from your partner or playmate, sharing your thoughts about pegging and anal play in each of the four categories. Then share your answers to look for overlap and to stimulate the ever-important communication!

Exciting

_____
_____
_____
_____
_____
_____
_____
_____
_____

Intriguing

_____
_____
_____
_____
_____
_____
_____
_____
_____

Scary

_____
_____
_____
_____
_____
_____
_____
_____
_____
_____

Concerns

_____
_____
_____
_____
_____
_____
_____
_____
_____
_____

Easing In

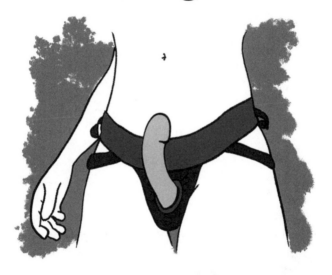

As anyone who's ever been fucked in the ass knows, you don't just drop your pants and *do it*. Unlike what is depicted in porn time and time again, anal sex takes time, finesse, ease. This is one of the reasons that for most couples it's not an every-time act, more like a special-occasions play.

Beyond needing to ease into anal play in general, any anal first timers out there will need a whole lot of prep work. We hesitate to call any of this foreplay, because your authors stand firmly in the "sex is sex is sex" camp, from the first sexual touch until the last. But we can call this fore-pegging-play without threat of any reprisal but an eye roll from our most jaded readers.

As with any other sex that isn't just a quick fuck, there's so much you can do that surrounds pegging without even strapping on (but you should feel free to strap on early and often.)

Communication

Really every chapter in this book could have a section with the header "communication." Every chapter in every book about sex in the world could. Talking about what you want to do, talking about how to do it, and talking about how it's going is truly the most valuable skill you can have as a sexual being.

Why is it so important here? Well, two reasons. First, the anus and rectum can be a bit finicky and are prone to tears and other issues. Second, in pegging, one party is wearing a dildo, and that dildo—as much as we would like it to—simply doesn't have nerve endings, so it's really like trying to lift a beer when your arm is asleep.

While we've addressed other sorts of communication earlier, now we're going to focus specifically on your pegging playtime.

Anyone who has spent any time in the BDSM community is likely familiar with the idea of safewords, which come in handy if you're playing with an intense fantasy or types of consensual play that mimic non-consent where you want to be able to fake-struggle and protest while still having a real way to stop the action if it goes too far.

If having a special word that means "stop" feels good to you, go for it. For the purposes of this book, though, we're going to assume you're just using language in a straightforward way, where "no" means "no," "yes" means "yes," and "please god fuck me harder I can't believe how amazing this feels" means just that.

Two things worth noting for those new to the pegging experience, though, are about disconnection and getting lost in the experience. For those getting pegged for the first time, especially if you are near a prostate orgasm, it can become an almost out-of-body experience, and it isn't unheard of for the peg-gee to go nonverbal here and there. We've both seen and experienced this. At the beginning of a session, the receiver should be able to communicate direction easily and effectively, giving tips of faster/slower, realignment, wait, etc. Once the real thrusting happens, though, sometimes all bets are off. As the pegger, we must remember that the cock sticking out of our bodies, while it may look incredibly realistic, doesn't give us the tactile sensation and feedback we would get from a nerve-connected appendage, and thus we need to rely on our partner for much of that feedback.

External Prostate Massage

If insertion isn't your thing just yet, there are ways to massage the prostate, and maybe even come to a prostate orgasm, using external play only. It's not the most direct stimulation, so it may not be as intense, but starting out slow and exploring all the options is a great way to get used to all of this. The perineum, otherwise known as the taint, is the area between the balls or vulva and the butthole. That little inch or so of flesh is usually soft enough to gently push up into to reach the prostate.

The prostate may also be massaged by gently rubbing the low belly area, below the belly button but above the pubic bone.

If the movement makes the person getting the massage feel as if they may have to pee, you're probably in the right spot. For men and women, we suggest trying to pee before and after sex, because when you're hitting the G-spot or the P-spot, knowing you don't have any pee in your system will alleviate that feeling of, "Oh no, I have to pee right now!" Your body is merely signaling to you that it's wrapped your urethra in a very solid grip. Peeing *after* sex is just good hygiene so no one gets a UTI (urinary tract infection).

Just as exploring the anus with a finger during a blowjob can add to the pleasure immensely, exploring testicular play and perineal massage during a blowjob can really kick it up a notch. Try using hands, fingers, a tongue, a toy, or any other safe object to help in this massage.

While perineal play and external prostate massage isn't actually pegging, it's a wonderful addition to your sexual repertoire and a great place to start your explorations. Even if you never actually do the whole pegging thing, we cannot recommend this type of play highly enough.

Spit Is Not Lube

Okay, so, for many of us who've exclusively had heterosexual sex with people who are very excited, the experience has involved the self-lubrication of a hungry vulva and vagina. (Not to call dentata to mind...) It's relevant, of course, that some vagina-havers don't get wet, and getting wet is not the sole determiner of interest. The point is, sometimes, in some situations that we may have experienced, after a little play outside, the inside gets much slicker and ready to take whatever we choose to put inside.

This is *not* the case, however, with the butt. We'll not take a stance on whether or not the butt was "designed" for sex, as we don't particularly think anything was "designed," nor should it matter. But the point is that the anus and rectum are not self-lubricating, and do their best, in fact, to keep stuff moving in the functional direction (out).

So, lube is going to be essential here. We'll go over a lot of different lubes and make suggestions in our Best Tools for the Job section later, but you definitely need lubrication.

And while we're on that subject, we're going to emphatically state a fact. Spit is not lube. Say it with us, folks:

Spit is not lube.

We don't care what you've seen in porn and how hot you may find it when someone spits on their hand and then slides right in. What you didn't see was the likelihood of a butt plug worn for hours prior, the lube-shooter filled with lube going up their rear, and the copious amounts of lube already in play before the spit even happens.

While we generally hesitate to tell anyone what to do, we're not going to hesitate here. Don't use spit as lube with anal sex. Just because it may sorta almost work for vaginal sex (but, really, don't use spit for vaginal sex either—lube exists for a reason, folks), doesn't mean it's a good idea for anal.

Anyway. We'll just say that folks who *do* use spit as lube for anal generally only do it once and we'll let you figure out why that is.

Now that you *have* lube, though, we don't recommend just lubing up the dildo and inserting. The reason that method can work with vulvas is because the lube enhances the natural lubricant already present, and they work together to make the experience as slick as possible. The anus is not self-lubricating and needs all the help it can get.

On Your Back

A great position to begin pegging, and one we recommend, is for the receiver to lie on their back and the giver to kneel between their legs. This isn't only for the actual act of pegging, but for much of the prep work. The reason for this is that eye contact can be incredibly important.

As much as we say in this book how important communication is (and don't think it isn't!), we also remember and acknowledge that communication isn't always easy, especially if you're doing something new or scary. Because of this, being able to look each other in the face can be the most valuable thing you can do for your exploration. We get into a bunch of fun options for positions later in the book, but when you are just starting out, this is a great beginner position.

Also, because your face isn't buried in a pillow, you're able to say things like "more," "less," "up," "down," and other specific communication of desires without them coming out as a muffled stream of consonants. You also tend to feel more empowered to say something when you can look at each other. And as the pegger, there's nothing clearer than a wince to tell you that maybe you should slow down and ask, "What's going on?"

It's important to clarify, though, that you shouldn't be reliant on body language versus actual human wordy language. Reading your partner's body language can sometimes end up creating a need to read their mind. While some playmates may be squirming in the throes of orgasmic ecstasy, others may be squirming to desperately get away. In this case, assumptions are not a great thing.

'Cuz, you know what happens when you assume? Asses are involved. And not in the good way.

Address the Anus

Okay, we've talked about it enough. Let's get right in there, shall we? Many men have little to no experience with anal sex, so it's important to take this in stages. You may jump through all of the prep stages and be silicone-balls-deep by the end of the night. Don't plan for that, though. Try to take every stage as it comes and decide together if you're ready to move on.

Before anything is inserted, a lubricated thumb run in circles around the anus can be wonderful.

There are so many nerve clusters in this small area that simple stimulation of it with only slight pressure can feel great. As you warm up the butthole, you'll notice it relax a bit as the blood flows to it. Once you feel this relaxing, talk with your partner to see how they feel about pressing forward.

We mean literally pressing forward, too. We're not inserting anything yet, just putting enough pressure on the anus to cause it to begin to open, ringing the proverbial doorbell. This will be the first moment where some discomfort can be felt, and if it is, go back to the circular rubbing and perhaps apply more lube.

An alternative or addition to finger-play is salad tossing/butt licking/analingus. Before we discuss this too much, we're going to mention that there are some germy/safety concerns here that we'll go into more later. If you and your partner wash regularly (and ideally, just before), you should be alright.

As with the fingering we mentioned above, salad tossing (no, we don't know why it's called that) isn't about jamming something into your partner's butt. It's about an overall pleasurable experience. A tongue moving in circles around the anus or pressing gently on it is also great preparatory work for eventual insertion, but as we've mentioned before, it can also be sex on its own. If the idea squicks you out a bit, try incorporating a dental dam or plastic wrap barrier between you and the butt in question. We highly recommend butt licking for you, for your partner, for America (insert country of origin or choice here, or whatevs).

Go for Insertion

There comes a time in every man's pegging life when he's been prepped thoroughly and is ready for having something in his ass. We don't recommend this moment being the pegging moment, though, as there's still a bit of warm-up and preparatory play. We know, we know, it feels like a lot, but it will make everything that much better in the long run, we promise.

Thankfully, most of us have come factory equipped with the best sex toys on the market: fingers. They make great toys because they're flexible, dexterous, and sensitive. The best a dildo can hope for is two out of those three. Fingers, on the other hand (to coin a phrase), are perfect.

As the finger-having person doing the inserting, you'll want to lube up, perhaps more than feels necessary, and insert slowly. Stimulation of the outer sphincter will allow it to open, and the inner sphincter should follow suit. Once you're inside the rectum, get the lay of the land, notice the smoothness of the walls, the openness of that vestibule. Then, when ready, curl your finger (or fingers—you can go at your own pace) back toward the top of the rectum (that is, point at the belly button from inside). Here's where you should feel the prostate.

Early in your playtime, it's going to be fairly small and subtle, feeling slightly like that squishy walnut. (Unless you have an enlarged prostate, which we talk about in our health section.) Some rubbing and caressing—not too firmly at this point—will cause the prostate to engorge and grow. Some will grow a little, some will grow a lot, but whatever its growth feels like, it will tighten.

The temptation now will be to start thrusting quickly. This is again a remnant of our collective porn obsession. Not everything is about being the biggest and the fastest, and the prostate produces different sensations in every body. The general rule of thumb for how to play with the prostate is very similar to the G-spot: that curled finger moving slightly deeper inside than the prostate and lightly tugging at it from behind. Some will like intense pressure on the prostate and little movement; others will enjoy strong back-and-forth rubbing. This is your time to experiment, communicate, and explore, as the information you learn here will greatly enhance your playtime.

As the receiver, you should pay close attention as fingers are inserted. What feelings are coming up? Pain? Pleasure? What happens with movement, with pressure against the walls of your rectum? How about when the fingers find your prostate? Are you feeling like you need to pee? Should you actually pee before you continue? (Yes. Full bladders rarely increase the sensation in prostate stimulation.) Do you prefer faster movements or pressure? Do you prefer more fingers or fewer? So much information can be gleaned from this exploratory session, and all of it is valuable.

Now, the fact that we called it an exploratory session doesn't mean you're going to graduate off to pegging and never return. Fingers and tongues are absolutely great for butt play and can always be incorporated into your sexy butt-play life. Sometimes you simply may not be ready, able, or interested in taking a dildo inside you, and that is alright.

And Now...Pegging

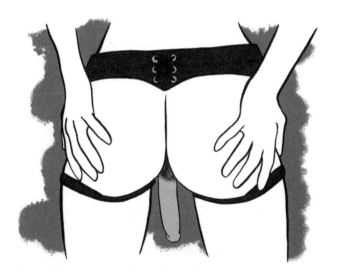

Alright. You've prepped, you've warmed up, you've lubed, you've strapped on, you've spread your legs and now let's get to some fucking pegging at last! As tempting as it might be for us to say "not so fast" or "there's one thing to remember first" because we enjoy trolling our readers, we've got literally nothing here. Now is your time, readers. Now, you peg.

In the next section we're going to regale you with a bunch of pegging positions, so for now we're going to talk about pegging itself in the most general way, while using the position of the pegger on their knees and the peggee on their back with their knees up. This is very close to the missionary position, though the two of you participating have likely swapped spots. This Corrupted Missionary Position takes the number-one spot on our list of best positions, in fact.

Insertion should, as with the fingers, be slow and steady, holding at times for as long as needed. You may need to take frequent breaks regardless of how many fingers may have made it inside, as a medium-sized dildo just *feels* different. Once you've inserted to the depth that the receiver enjoys, it's time to try some thrusting. Go slow and steady, keeping eye contact and conversation the entire time.

It's a good rule of thumb to let the receiver dictate the entire process this first time, giving clearance for speed changes and depth changes. After a while, the receiver may be overcome by the sensation and defer to the giver, but our advice is to still take this slow and make changes very gradually.

As the prostate orgasm is rather elusive, especially at first, and ejaculation is uncommon from pegging alone, the act doesn't really have a clearly defined end and often will simply continue until one or both of the participants decide to cease pegging.

What of the Penis?

We haven't talked much about the penis, as it's not really involved too much in the whole pegging experience. Sure, it *can* be, but it doesn't really need to be.

Very possibly, the peggee's dick won't be hard or will be semi-hard. As many people have been socialized to believe that a lack of erection means a lack of enjoyment, we want to swat this idea down immediately. First, regardless of pegging, erections can be affected by so many different things: stress, medication, exhaustion, illness, or simply the whims of the great God of Erections, forever may He rise. Second, especially in new-to-pegging people, the body has re-routed much of the blood it would normally be using to stay hard toward the butt, as the prostate engorges and the area becomes more sensitive, thus leaving little extra to keep hard.

Cooper will be the first to tell you that he's rarely hard during pegging. We're not sure if it's an explanabrag that he pegs a lot, or an attempt to make you feel better, but either way, we're mentioning it here.

Another thing of note is that, if you're chasing the prostate orgasm, you really ought to just leave that dick alone. (We considered a "Hey! Teacher..." Pink Floyd joke here, but it made us uncomfy.) Why shouldn't you play with your penis during pegging or prostate play? Well, we mean, you *can*, because you can do anything you want, but as the prostate orgasm is elusive and likes to send you down any off-ramp it can, nothing deflects it quite like an ejaculatory orgasm.

And as those of us who've ejaculated in the past know, we experience significant fatigue immediately after at the least, but also often an overwhelming bodily sensation that we may never need to ejaculate again. This is nature's way of getting us to calm the fuck down. So, if we shoot a load, the spirit may be willing but the body may be weak and the prostate orgasm will continue to elude us.

All this said, many men really enjoy penile stimulation during pegging, even without erection. If your goal is not a first-time prostate orgasm, feel free to grab that cock, as we continue to subscribe to the "you do you" ethos.

Best Pegging Positions

For decades now, in grocery store checkout lines, bold headlines on various magazine covers have promised to "drive him wild" or "spice up the bedroom" with their sex-position guides. Well, this isn't your momma's *Cosmo* magazine, nor are we going to bullshit you and assume you can hold your partner upside down in the shower while you fuck and not kill both yourself and your partner in the process. These are fun positions, but we don't want any of them to be impossible. They may still require a good amount of stretching to master, so limber up, drink some water, and prepare your body for a good fucking workout.

We did try to get creative with silly position names though, because that's half the fun. We use terms like top, bottom, giver, receiver, pegger, peggee, fucker, fuckee, penetrator, and penetrated throughout as they make sense within the positions.

CORRUPTED MISSIONARY

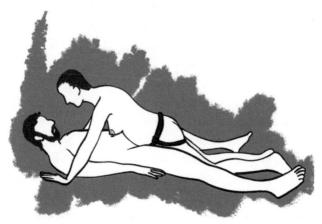

Description: The peggee is lying on their back, legs open to either side, and the pegger is lying on top of them between their legs. Partners are face to face.

Advantages: If you want the closeness of a lot of skin-on-skin contact, the connection of eye contact, and a generally more loving and romantic position, this might be the right fit for you.

Potential challenges: Bigger chests and bellies make this position harder and sometimes uncomfortable, so the size of the bodies at play may be something to consider.

Best tools for the job: A long, narrow, and firm toy would work best for this position, or use a wedge to boost the butt up in the air a few inches for ease of entry (we go over wedges and their helpfulness in the Best Tools for the Job chapter).

HOT DIGGITY DOG

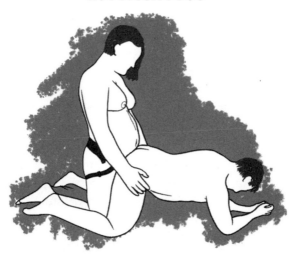

Description: The peggee is on their hands and knees, with the pegger kneeling behind them for rear entry.

Advantages: This is a good beginning-to-peg position because pegging can be a very vulnerable situation for the person being penetrated. Sometimes they can feel shy. They might not want eye contact with their partner and might rather focus on some inanimate object like a pillow or the wall to clear their head.

Potential challenges: Resting half of your weight on your hands is hard on the wrists and can be physically exhausting (as anyone who has tried to plank will know). Often in the "doggy-style" position, the peggee's arms will give out or tire and they will have to rest on their elbows or chest. This actually helps raise the butt up at a different angle and could be a good thing, but be mindful of arm strength and stamina.

Best tools for the job: A great tool for this position is a "doggy strap," which is a padded strap to put under the hips of the person being penetrated. It gives the pegger something to hold onto that isn't flesh (some people are delicate and bruise if you hold their love handles or thighs too tightly). As stated before, this position can be a little strenuous, so a wedge placed under the peggee's hips could be very helpful.

HAPPY BABY

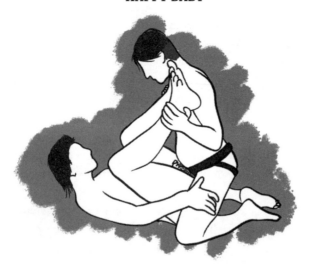

Description: The peggee is on their back with their legs up in the air over their head. The pegger is kneeling at the base of their body or resting their chest against the back of the bottom's legs.

Advantages: The pegger can rest their body against the back of their partner's legs, which can add a level of control for the person being pegged, as they can push the pegger back or pull them in deeper by moving their legs.

Potential challenges: This is an incredibly vulnerable position. The peggee is really putting everything out there in a balls-out kind of manner, literally. Not for the faint of heart, it's also a pretty good stretch and some folks who aren't super flexible might not be able to manage it (or for very long, anyway).

Best tools for the job: Since the ass will be on full display, any toy would most likely work, but a long, narrow, and firm toy will be the easiest to maneuver. Penetration will be deeper if the pegger literally gets on top of their partner's legs, so a shorter, curved-upward toy might be preferred.

COWBOY

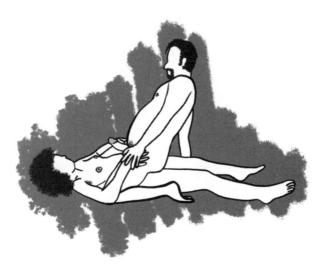

Description: The peggee is on top, riding their partner while facing them.

Advantages: The person being pegged is in control in this position. They get to ease their body down onto the dildo, control the depth and speed, as well as control how they ride the cock. They can lean over their partner for closer contact or kissing, and they can still feel like the fucker while simultaneously being fucked (because positionally they're looking down).

Potential challenges: This position can be hard on the legs and knees. Additionally, if the pegger and peggee's body sizes differ by a significant amount, it can push the bounds of flexibility.

Best tools for the job: A dildo with an upward curve works well in this position, especially if the peggee plans to lean over their partner for smooches. A toy that is very basic, straight up and down, would also work well, so they can ease onto the toy without trying to work the angle.

REVERSE COWBOY

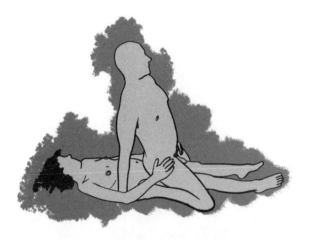

Description: The peggee is on top, riding their partner with their back turned to them.

Advantages: Similar to the regular "cowboy" position, the peggee gets to control everything. This position just offers another angle, less eye contact, and a way to lean over and rest on their hands or hold onto their partner's legs if they get tired.

Potential challenges: This position can be hard on the legs and knees, and can also feel a bit like doing the splits sideways.

Best tools for the job: An upward curve isn't ideal for this position unless the toy is worn upside down. A softer, bendable toy is best, as this position can really bend the toy downward.

LOTUS

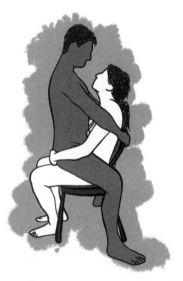

Description: The pegger is seated, and their partner is sitting in their lap, facing them.

Advantages: Great position for peggers with disabilities, who use a wheelchair, or who are injured and need to be seated during sex. Also a great position for the peggee to control depth, speed, and angle.

Potential challenges: Can be tiring for the peggee's legs due to bouncing up and down, with legs either bent on the side of a chair/couch/bed, or standing with legs on either side of a chair. Imagine an intense squat workout, but you get off at the end. It's a lot of work, but it's fun work. This is a very intimate position as both parties are face to face, chest to chest, and crotch to crotch.

Best tools for the job: A thigh harness might be a good choice for the pegger. A toy that is very basic, straight up and down, would work well so that the peggee can ease onto the toy at their discretion.

LAP DANCE

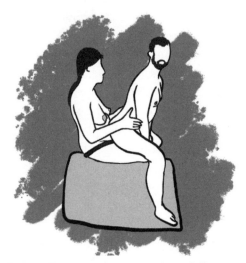

Description: The pegger is seated, and their partner is sitting in their lap with their back to them.

Advantages: The peggee can really grind on the crotch of the pegger and go to town fucking themselves *and* their partner. Similar to the Lotus, this is a great position for folks with disabilities, who use a wheelchair, or who are injured and need to be seated during sex.

Potential challenges: It is also quite the squat workout, so the peggee should prepare themselves for wobbly legs after.

Best tools for the job: An upward curve isn't ideal for this position unless the toy is worn upside down. A softer, bendable toy or straight up and down toy is best for this position.

STANDING SHOWER

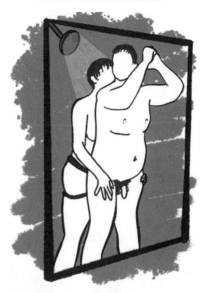

Description: Both partners are standing in the shower. The peggee is braced against the wall, legs spread open, with the pegger standing behind them, fucking from behind.

Advantages: This position leads itself to super easy cleanup for folks who may be squeamish around the idea of anal sex including any kind of poop. We get into that in our section on hygiene, but it's really not as big of an issue as one might assume. However, if it is a concern, shower sex is squeaky clean.

Potential challenges: This position can be tricky for folks with a big height discrepancy. Also, folks who try this out may need extra lube because it can get washed away from the shower (water is *not* lube—in fact it seems to make things less slippery) and using too much lube can pose a danger if the shower floor gets slippery. Use caution and be careful with this one.

Best tools for the job: A harnessless dildo might be a great addition to this position if the pegger doesn't want to get their harness wet (leather would be a big concern here). Despite the name, harnessless dildos don't stay in perfectly without a harness, as we've mentioned, but the pegger can help hold it in place, and this adds a level of penetration play for them as well.

OVER THE MOON

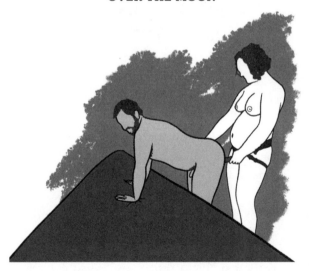

Description: The peggee is bent over the side of the bed, feet planted on the floor, legs spread, with their partner standing behind them, taking them from behind.

Advantages: This could be a fun kinky roleplay position. Maybe the pegger is an officer, and their partner is getting cuffed (then fucked). Maybe the pegger is a demanding professor who wants to give their student a few spankings before taking their ass to teach them a lesson.

Potential challenges: The height of the bed and the length of the pegger's legs are going to determine if this is a comfortable or even possible position. If the pegger's butt needs to be propped up a bit, consider getting a wedge or a couple of firm pillows to tuck under them.

Best tools for the job: A fun addition could be a pair of cuffs or some rope to tie the peggee's hands behind them if you want to go the kinky route.

MASSAGE TABLE

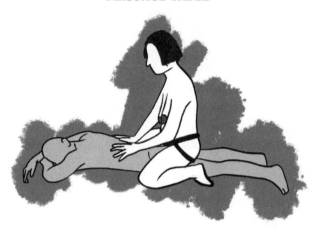

Description: The bottom is lying down flat on their stomach with the top sitting on their butt, as if to give a massage, entering from behind. Bonus points for rubbing the bottom's back, shoulders, and butt.

Advantages: This can be a very caring, generous, and thoughtful position. Most folks love a massage, and folks who have some level of trepidation when it comes to being penetrated might have a lot of nervous energy to expel. A great way to get relaxed and in the mood for play.

Potential challenges: As the pegger will be on their knees for this position, it can be rough on the knees, and legs have a tendency to fall asleep if tucked under one's body for too long.

Best tools for the job: Get a good massage oil that can double as an anal lubricant. Oil isn't great for vaginal health, so we don't suggest it for PIV sex, but it does work well for anal.

SPOON FORKING

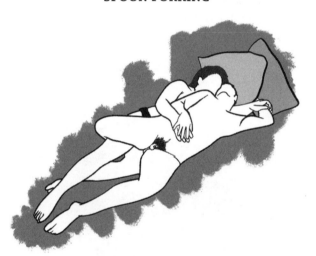

Description: Pegging in the spoon position. The fucker is lying behind the fuckee, penetrating them while cuddling.

Advantages: As a comfy, lazy position, this one can be nice and cuddly for both players. Great for chilly winters when you just want to snuggle up under a warm blanket but still want to get your fuck on.

Potential challenges: This position could be a little difficult because the pegger can't see where their toy is going and has to feel their way around under the covers.

Best tools for the job: A nice cotton underwear harness is going to be the most comfortable option for wearing to sleep. The wearer could even just take the toy out and keep it on if they're too tired to change.

DOUBLE TROUBLE

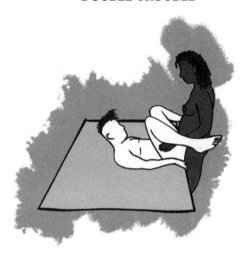

Description: The bottom is lying on their back, ass off the edge of the bed, knees up to their chest, with the top standing between their legs. This position gives the top the ability to give a handjob or blowjob at the same time as pegging.

Advantages: This can be a very sexy position as the peggee gets treated to anal as well as penis stimulation.

Potential challenges: While all that sensation may seem super appealing, it may also be a little overwhelming for some. This position may also be a complex move, flexibility-wise, as the pegger needs to be pretty flexible to do a blowjob while pegging (a handjob while pegging shouldn't be difficult, though). The pegger should read their partner's body language and communicate throughout to check in. Sometimes someone being pegged won't get an erection because blood flow is headed to the rear. This doesn't mean they aren't turned on, but that there's not enough blood to fill the erection and the prostate area.

Best tools for the job: The toy should be long enough that if the top bends over to try to go down on their partner, it doesn't just pop out.

Aftercare

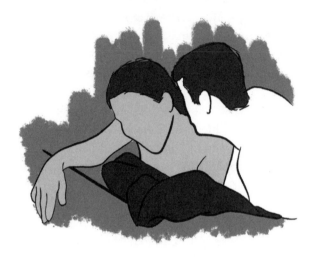

Pegging can be quite intense and sometimes over-whelming for both parties involved, especially in the early days of the act. With this in mind, we recommend considering and planning some extended aftercare.

What is aftercare? Well, the current use of the term seems to have originated in the BDSM community recognizing the amount of come-down time required after a particularly intense scene, or the need for realignment to return to "normal" after being in specific roles. While it's true that BDSM more often requires strong aftercare moments, it's important to recognize that all sex could use a bit of aftercare, if only to reconnect and decompress. This is especially true if you have children to get back to, as the shift from intimacy to parenting can be jarring.

Planning and building your aftercare into your sexy time will only enhance the experience for both of you. Here are some good ideas to help ease you into the rest of your night or day—maybe you're into pegging first thing in the morning, and who are we to judge?

* Sharing a bath or shower by candlelight, helping to wash one another.
* If solitary showers are your happy place, taking a relaxing shower alone may be your cup of tea.
* Wrapping up in a large blanket like a burrito and cuddling.
* Stretching out any sore muscles with some light, in-bed yoga moves.
* A mutual massage, taking turns and giving each other a good rubdown with some sensual-smelling massage oils.
* Sharing some nice chocolate or sugary treats.
* Taking a nice cuddly nap or sleeping together after a scene can do wonders.
* Watching a familiar, feel-good movie together.
* Hydration is a must. Pegging is a great workout, so make sure to get enough water!

After you've taken this base time to relax, good old communication comes into play. This is a great time to chat about the experience you both just shared. What did you enjoy? What felt great, and what not so great? What could use some work? What would you like to do again? Would you like to keep going at the same rate, go faster, or go slower next time? You don't have to go as far as ranking the experience by holding up cards, but the more you process together, the better your next time will be, especially if you experienced something far to the ends of the great-to-horrible spectrum.

And it's worth reminding yourself that aftercare will look different to everybody. If our list seems full of things you have no interest in doing, that's alright. Aftercare is a concept, a state of mind, not a specific act or type of act. All that matters is that it makes you and your partner feel good.

Health Benefits

Again reminding y'all of our "we are not doctors" ethos, let's talk briefly about the physiological health benefits of anal play in men and prostate-havers.

As Cooper loves to overshare in our class, we thought it only proper that we do the same here. He has prostatitis III. Thankfully this is the annoying one of the prostatitis family and not one of the "gonna try hard to kill you with cancer" ones. Prostatitis III is very common in people who have desk jobs and sit for most of their days. It manifests as an inflamed prostate that leads to chronic pain. It's also referred to as CPPS, Chronic Pelvic Pain Syndrome.

For him, it manifests as chronic pain up and down his thighs and lower back, and on the worst days it feels as though his balls are in a vise grip and causes him to look back fondly on the day in sixth grade when a "friend" kneed him in the balls because said "friend" had wondered what would happen.

Because of this condition, Cooper has had his prostate examined multiple times, likely more so than most other men in their early forties. In one visit with his proctologist, he mentioned he was into prostate massage and asked if that might do anything to help.

The doctor replied, "Well, prostate massage is something that we do for people with advanced prostatitis and other prostate issues."

Then, always a stickler, Cooper asked point-blank if prostate massage would be beneficial for his CPPS and the doctor said, rather cagily: "Well, I can't tell you that your prostate play will help. I can tell you that sometimes we do this to help."

We agree that this is his way of saying without saying yes, playing with your prostate *does* help.

The field of research surrounding the health benefits of pleasurable prostate stimulation is very narrow and woefully underfunded, as it is with most any pleasure-based sex discussion. This is why no sciencey folk are out to find the G-spot when so many of us can literally show them where it is located.

Every once in a while, a study will come out that concludes something like regular masturbation leads to a lowered risk of prostate cancer and the media pounces on it because they find it funny, and cranky old people start talking about thinking about the children, and it's dropped.

What this mostly suggests, though, is frequent prostatic fluid expulsion, be it from masturbation to ejaculation, more traditional sex, or rubbing the prostate until the genie comes out, has a more than 0 percent chance of keeping your prostate healthy longer. And you know what? More than zero is pretty awesome.

Safety and Comfort

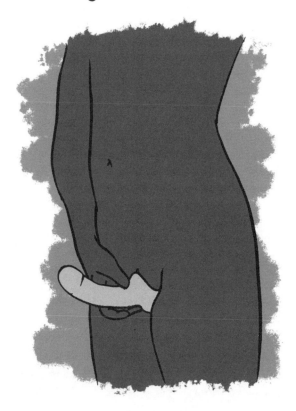

Does It Hurt?

Some of the most common questions we get asked when it comes to anal sex (for both men and women) are about pain and discomfort. "I have never been able to do anal. It hurts too much!" someone will say, dismissing the entire act from one bad experience (or many, unfortunately).

Generally speaking, if there is any pain, something is wrong. There may always be a little bit of discomfort in the beginning because your body is not used to things going into "out" holes. It takes time to adjust and for your body to get comfortable with that sensation. It takes time for your brain to rewire from "Ouch, things don't go there!" to "Oh, this is hot." Often, if there's discomfort, your body isn't relaxed enough, you're not using enough lube, or the object that you're trying to insert may be a little bit too big. And this goes for all sex acts: if it hurts, take a step back and evaluate the situation.

The anal canal actually has two sphincters. The outer one is voluntary, meaning you can actually move it. When you're clenching your butt cheeks or doing a pelvic floor Kegel exercise (let's all do one for good measure right now. Deep breath in, clench! Exhale, release! Nice.), you are moving your voluntary sphincter. There is also an involuntary one just inside the voluntary one, which is not as easy to control. To relax the second sphincter, your body actually has to be relaxed. If you are tense, that sphincter will be tensed up. Pushing through the tightness of it may cause discomfort until your body gets used to the sensation.

If you experience sharp pain or a tearing sensation, you should definitely stop to make sure you aren't injured or aren't going to further injure yourself by continuing.

Body language ends up being a huge component of pegging. Tensing, squirming away, going stiff, a sharp intake of breath, a facial grimace, or even just a silent partner can all be signs that things aren't feeling great. A pause may be in order to establish how they're doing. Frequent check-ins are always a great way to prevent pain and discomfort.

The shape and size of your toy is also going to make a difference. There's a saying that "Your eyes are bigger than your stomach" when it comes to ordering too much food and then overeating and being uncomfortable or not being able to finish what you started. Similarly, we like to say, "Your eyes are bigger than your ass." Sometimes folks will find a toy similar to their own penis size and assume that must be the right fit for them. Sometimes a warped sense of toxic masculinity tells them that they can (and should) take on more than their body is able to. It's like they are gunning to earn their Take It Like A Man badge of honor.

Always remember that being uncomfortable is not sexy. It's not fun, it's rarely enjoyable (unless you're kinky like that), and it can ruin a scene for both you and your partner. For the sake of both of you, take things slow.

Start anal exploration with just fingers. If the idea of that freaks you out, wear gloves. At the very least, clip your fingernails and file for any sharp edges. We'll go over hygiene in our next section, so you'll figure out ways to lessen any yucky feelings you may have over this act. If needed, put on a glove (or have a partner put one on), lube up a finger or two, and figure that ass out! What feels good? What feels weird? It probably all feels weird in the beginning, but give it time.

When exploring the ass, it is essential that you are already aroused. Feeling around for your prostate when you are not turned on is going to feel like a medical exam, and probably not in a fun, kinky way. The prostate enlarges when the body is turned on, so it's much easier to find, and it won't feel nearly as clinical or un-sexy if you've already started foreplay with a partner.

Begin with just a single finger. Play outside of the anus. Give the area a little massage. Sit with that feeling, so to speak. Enter the anus tentatively and gently. Again, feel around like it's part of a massage. It's nice to incorporate this kind of play into oral sex, as it adds a little extra sensation to an already fun, seductive act.

Once that feels comfortable, graduate to two fingers. Then add in a small or "entry-level" butt plug when you feel ready. A good way to practice getting used to anal play in general is to wear a butt plug while you have other kinds of sex. Wear it while doing your favorite sex act. Like Pavlov's dog, you'll begin to associate the feeling of anal sensation with hot sexiness (it may even make *you* drool too!).

Once you get past the fingers or small butt plug stage, try a slender dildo on for size. We like to recommend trying it out solo first so you know what to expect and can go at exactly the right pace for you, but it's entirely understandable if you would like to experiment with your partner first. Make sure that your partner is well-versed in your body language or check in with them regularly. Anal sex can be overwhelming, so take your time.

Going too hard, too fast, and with too much girth and not enough lube are the biggest issues with pain and discomfort. Due to the sphincter muscles having to stretch so much to accommodate a toy, girth is a much more important factor than length. When picking out a toy, do a mental comfort check of both girth and length.

And on the topic of lube: Use a lot. Use more than you would think. Use lube intended specifically for anal play. Use super-slippery silicone or thick gel lube that won't soak into your skin in two thrusts. Then use some more, and reapply often. We have a common saying that the main tenets of anal sex are 1. communication and 2. lubrication. Silicone lube is great for anal play because a little goes a long way and it stays slippery for a long time.

Hugs, Not Drugs

If you're feeling nervous about pain during anal play, it might seem obvious to just cover up that anxiety with an emotional painkiller of some kind. We want to dissuade you of that knee-jerk reaction. Firstly, most of us aren't making good decisions when we're three sheets to the wind in a bottle of whiskey or several puffs on the vape pen. Whenever we're doing something new, especially something that feels scary to us, we should be wide awake both physically and mentally.

The other painkiller many newbies to anal will often cling to is a desensitizing cream for the anus like Anal-Eaze. We can tell you, though, that using a product like this is really setting yourself up for a potentially unsexy morning after. Drugs and alcohol *can* lessen pain and anxiety during the sex itself, but as they begin to wear off, you'll start to feel any damage you may have done. Anal-Eaze, or any other kind of desensetizer (like throat numbing spray), as well as the aforementioned alcohol and drugs, can keep you pain-free in the moment, but only by masking the pain that you, perhaps, should have been feeling.

It's like when you get all Novacained up at the dentist and then try to eat McDonalds on the way home. (Just us?) You wind up chewing the hell out of your cheek, tongue, and lip because you can't feel them, and dribbling your Orange Fanta all down your chest. Well, imagine your cheek, tongue, and lip are your asshole. Or...maybe...hrm.

The bottom line is that if you can't feel damage as it's happening, you won't work to prevent it. While anal sex may have some discomfort at the very beginning, it's not supposed to *hurt*, and if it does, it's likely because you're actually damaging your butt! Vigorous anal sex can cause anal fissures or micro tears in the sensitive skin around the anus, and in the rectum itself. In the short term you can count on these being incredibly painful while they heal, but in the long term it's even worse. These fissures will turn into scar tissue. Since scars don't have as much elasticity as regular skin, it will be harder and harder to stretch the sphincter in any significant way, meaning your future anal sex has greater potential to cause anal fissures, which then scar, which then tighten. A regular snowball effect of pain and discomfort.

This is all a big and scary (and necessary) way of saying that if your anal sex hurts, you might be doing it wrong, and it is very important for you to realize and know that in the moment rather than the following morning. In addition, if you've managed to numb yourself up enough that you can't feel pain, doesn't it follow that you're depriving yourself of the pleasure happening at that moment as well?

Speaking of drugs, some folks, especially in gay communities, have long been using poppers, a drug which will get someone high within seconds and can help to relax the anal sphincter muscles. Other names it goes by are amyl nitrate, butyl nitrite, video-head cleaner, rush, liquid gold, jungle juice, and leather cleaner. It seems like there's a new slang word made up for it daily. Recreational use of poppers became super popular in the gay bar and club scene because it gave users a fearless energy around anal and oral sex. The user feels like they can take on anything and everything, throat or ass. Folks who have experience with this drug may think it's the best thing under the sun, but we do not recommend it for folks just starting out. As we've stated, an inebriated ass may not be able to feel pain at the moment, but it sure will the next morning. There has also been some troubling research into the use of poppers connected to losing eyesight, intense headaches, sinus problems, and allergic reactions, so be careful out there folks!

We do feel rather drug shamey at the moment, so we'd like to say that this isn't DARE, and we're not trying to tell you *not* to do drugs. Our sole focus is protecting your precious butts so you can have more awesome buttsex. And if telling you not to do drugs in *this specific instance* will help us do that, we're gonna tell you not to do drugs.

When you're not having anal sex, you go ahead and do all the drugs you want so long as they're not hurting you or others.

At the risk of sounding all "get high on life, man" there are some things you can do that will have some of the same effects as the aforementioned drugs. For instance, if you like the idea of the anal and sphincter area feeling a little numb but still registering both pain and pleasure, you can get that with a vibrator. Have you ever held a strong buzzy vibrator in your hand for a while? Your whole hand will begin to feel numb. This holds true for your butt. While most any vibe will do the work, you'll likely want to go for the big guns in a wand-type vibrator held against the anus and perineum (remember the perineum, or taint, is the area between the anus and the balls). This will cause that whole area to numb up a little bit for a little while. This will, more importantly, also relax those muscles, which will naturally allow the anus to dilate and make penetration far easier.

Leading up to anal playtime, a massage can help you relax thoroughly. (We do recommend you offer to reciprocate—it's just selfish to be a massage hog.) A back massage can easily move into a butt massage, which can then become a butthole massage. For a little added fun here, slide his cock and balls back between his legs so you can stroke with a well-lubed hand while playing with his butt.

As always, playing it safer here will allow you to play again and again.

Do You Dig My Flare?

On that note, one more thing about safe butt play.

A flared base may be the most important phrase ever when it comes to things being inserted in butts. We've spoken a lot about using fingers and dildos in harnesses. Both of those things have the benefit of being attached to, well, people, and thus unlikely to be lost in the caverns of the rectum. Horrifying, we know.

We've all seen the medical shows where doctors joke about the many things they've found in people's butts and how the patient usually claims to have tripped and fallen on it so as not to admit the simple fact that a *lot* of people like having a *lot* of things put into their butts. Well, this doesn't just happen on TV, it happens in real life, too. And unfortunately, it's not usually as funny and sometimes requires surgery to remove the foreign object.

This is why there's a common saying at sex toy stores and among sex educators. In a fun sing-songy voice, we like to say, "Without a base, without a trace!" and "Without flare, keep it outta there!" We like to rhyme—it helps folks remember important things.

Due to the arrangement of your sphincter muscles, and the fact that they're mostly designed to keep you from pooping when you don't want to poop, your butthole can be a little like a vacuum, sucking things right in, if given the opportunity. This is the number-one reason we do not suggest doing like the porn shows and shoving produce or other household things up your bum.

Anal toys, and most dildos, are designed with flared bases that are wider than the widest point of the toy, and many will dip down to their thinnest point right before the base. This encourages your outer sphincter to clamp down just before the flare and have the base rest against your asshole, holding it in place and keeping it from disappearing inside. Toys not made for anal play, like bullet vibes and baby carrots, do not have the flare and are prone to vanishing.

One more thing. Should something disappear inside you or your partner, don't panic and call 911 right away. The bottom line is that you already have a mechanism for getting things out of you. It's called pooping and you know how to do it. So, squat or sit on the toilet and gently push. Most of the time whatever went up will come back down.

The reason for all the above concern is when something changes positions, or has extra ridges or...action figure hands...keeping it from returning. Seriously, don't shove action figures up your butt. Neither the figures nor your butt will likely be happy with the result.

If you find yourself at this point, there are really two options: your partner going on a finger-based fishing expedition, or going to the hospital to see where that toy has wandered. It's always going to be preferable to have a partner essentially have to fist you to get a lost toy out of your rectum than to have a doctor or nurse do so at the hospital. But anal fisting is not for the weak of heart (or ass), and no one wants their first experience with it to be in an emergency situation.

So, yeah, always use toys with a flared base, and *really*, don't ever put anything in your butt that wasn't specifically designed to be safe to go in your butt. We care about your butt and only want what's best for it.

Shit Happens

Well, it does!

It's time to have the talk. We know you've been thinking about it. One of the most common fears around anal sex, across the gender spectrum, is poop. Will I have to deal with it? Will anal make me feel like I have to poop? Will there be a huge mess? Is it going to get on me, my partner, or my sheets? Do I have to make sure there's no poop in my body to play?

Take a deep breath, and we'll get through this together.

Yes, your body, right now, probably has poop in it. Don't worry—that's normal. It means you're human. As they say, everybody poops. And shit, as they say, happens. But you really don't have to worry as much as you probably are.

At a certain point, if you enjoy pegging and anal play or really want to try both, you sort of have to recognize the fact that you probably will, at some point in your anal exploration, get shit on you. Get over it. There's shit inside you and it comes out your butt.

To lessen your fears, we're here to tell you that poop (sounds friendlier that way, doesn't it?) doesn't become an issue as frequently as you might think. Poop doesn't just sit around in your rectum all day. It hangs out in your intestines. If you make a point to poop at some point earlier in the day (or Sunday morning if you're blasphemous) then it will be flushed out of your rectum and colon by the time you're inviting someone inside.

That said, you should pay attention to your body here, as some people have more frequent bowel movements than others or have fewer pre-poop warning signals. But be smart about it. If you know that a big latte or Taco Bell or other things make you need to spend significant amounts of time sitting on the toilet, maybe don't eat or drink those things in your pre-pegging time. After, sure. Make yourself a Taco Bell feast with lattes all around to celebrate that prostate orgasm.

Now we know that saying you should get over poop isn't *really* helpful, and it's likely going to have enough societal stigma and shame surrounding it that it might take some time to actually get over it. Don't worry—there are a few things that you can do to clean yourself out or mitigate the poop problem.

Enemas

Some people who are new to anal play can really go around the bend on the cleanliness issue and buy out their local Rite-Aid's supply of enemas. Though those items can be helpful occasionally to flush yourself out, be careful because you can really overdo it.

If you are giving yourself an enema every single time you have sex or any time you're preparing for sex, it can cause an imbalance of the natural good bacteria in your colon. All that water sloshing around in the solids section can make a lot of people feel nauseous as well. Not to mention the bloating and the fullness. If you don't manage to expel all the enema water before you get to the anal sex, you're just pushing that further and further inside and sloshing it around. And for...stuff...it's not supposed to go backwards. It's really a one-way trip.

Enemas can actually make your anal play (or the period directly after it) messier when you don't get all the water out. The last thing you want is to be, say, in line at the grocery store and have some of that water come tumbling out. Or you sneeze and make a mess. Or your attempt to mitigate the problem of poop actually leads to a poopy-watery mixture coming out during the very anal sex you're trying to keep clean.

We aren't saying to never use enemas. Gay porn stars swear by them! Professionals in the anal sex field will use enemas, not eat for a solid day before a performance, and wear a butt plug to stretch out for *hours* to prep for a scene. But unless you're racking up cash for a porn shoot, we happen to think all of that prep is a little *extra*.

Some couples enjoy enemas as part of their sexy pre-gaming and play. It can even be part of a fun medical roleplay fetish, but do it in moderation. For comfort and medical reasons, never use cold or soapy water, and give yourself a good long while to finish expelling all the water before it's time for the sex.

For an enema-like sensation without the entire up-the-bum experience, invest in a bidet. There are numerous styles out there that screw right onto your toilet, can be installed in minutes, and aren't that costly. They do the job of cleaning up the outer anal area much better than toilet paper ever can, and get into the deep crevices better than a basic shower will. Brace yourself with these—if you don't splurge on a heated bidet, that shock of cold water can be quite the eye-opening experience.

Shaving may also be on your agenda. In general, a shaved or trimmed area makes things easier to clean, but we know as well as any how hard it is to shave your own butt crack. Even the most practiced yogi is going to find that flexibility a bit difficult. Having a partner (or trusted friend, or wax-wielding professional esthetician) help you out with hair removal may be the right course if you can't reach the area easily. To make hair removal more comfortable, we don't recommend harsh hair-removal chemicals (like Nair), since the area is so sensitive that the chemicals could burn like hell. Use a new razor, a soft touch, and hair conditioner or shaving gel to help clean the area of hair.

Know though, that once you start shaving, you kind of have to keep it up. Every teenage girl has to come to terms with this realization once she starts shaving her legs—there's no going back. Stubble, especially between one's butt cheeks, is annoying at best and a downright horrible, itchy, pain-in-the-literal-ass at worst.

If shaving isn't your thing, you can still get squeaky clean with a full butt-bush of hair.

Mitigation of the Mind

Now, even if you can acknowledge and be ostensibly okay with the fact that shit happens, you may still want to do some mitigation in the moment. Two easy methods to keep your mind at ease are:

1. Use black condoms on the pegging dildo. This doesn't get rid of poop, but sure makes it much more difficult to get a glimpse of and get in your head about.
2. Have a dark towel nearby. The towel can be used to clean any issues and can become a wrap for the dildo post-sex.

Some of us feel much more comfortable knowing that we will be the ones to take care of our own poop, and pulling a soiled condom off or wrapping the dildo in a towel allows us to take charge and disappear into the bathroom to clean up.

A point of note: Most black condoms are made out of latex, so if you have a latex allergy, this strategy may not work for you.

If you can't get out of your head, it will negatively affect your sexual experience. Not being able to focus on your pleasure makes for a difficult time in facilitating an orgasm.

Have wet wipes on hand, on the side table, in the bathroom, or wherever it is clever for personal cleanup. Anal sex can be a bit of a lubey mess. Silicone lube especially is hard to just wipe off. Water-based lube will dry up or soak into the skin eventually, but silicone is a lot more like oil in that it stays slippery even in the presence of water. Great for shower sex and long-lasting, but messy as all get out. Wet wipes can help to clean off lubed-up hands, so you're not slipping and sliding all over your partner's body (unless you're into that).

The reason we harp on the idea that shit will happen, though, is that if you go into your pegging exploration knowing that fact, and you have a good relationship with your partner, it really doesn't matter. To stay out of your head and mitigate the butt shame you may feel, implement any of the suggestions we've given above. All of these suggestions are not meant to prevent a moment involving poop, but to be an easy way to get rid of it immediately, should it happen. Condoms on toys, towels nearby, and of course, gloves.

The Glory of Gloves

There are few things in the world smoother than surgical gloves covered in lube. We will go so far as to recommend wearing gloves of the latex or nitrile variety even without concerns about poop or health because they provide an amazingly smooth experience. Don't buy the cheapest ones you can, as they'll likely be loose-fitting and break easily.

We recommend nitrile as they're available in many different colors and sizes and they avoid any concern about latex allergies. Believe us, you don't want to learn you have a latex allergy from a reaction inside your rectum. Order one size smaller than you think you'll need, as this will be the most formfitting.

Nitrile is also great for fingering if you have anything longer than very close-cut fingernails, as the nitrile will cushion and help prevent any horrifying fingernail-butt fissures. If you have *really* long nails, though, you run the risk of puncturing the glove. You can try putting cotton balls in the fingertips of the gloves, but we really recommend shorter fingernails if you're going to do a lot of finger-in-a-butt play.

Washing and Sterilizing Toys

Good hygiene isn't just about you, but also about your toys. We always recommend using condoms on your toys, but when those condoms come off, the toy should still be thoroughly cleaned to prevent bacteria buildup and to minimize the chance of STI transmission.

This transmission is less of an issue if you are monogamous and fluid bonded with your partner. (That is, if it's cool if your bodily fluids go inside their body, and vice versa.) But if you are non-monogamous or do any sharing of toys, this sterilization is essential, as it has been discovered that the HPV virus can remain on silicone toys even after a thorough soap and water scrubbing for up to twenty-four hours. Shocked? So were we!

Before we get too deep into how to wash and sterilize, we'd like to note that we *exclusively* recommend silicone toys for pegging. For other activities, stainless steel, glass, and pyrex toys are also excellent, but they can be dangerous for pegging due to the lack of sensation for the giver and, thus, the chance of pushing too hard against areas that really don't have a lot of give. Silicone on the other hand, has decent-to-good give, and is not porous. It is also *fully sterilizable*. We go a little bit deeper into the subject of toy material in the Best Tools for the Job section later.

Did you know that you can clean your toys in the dishwasher? Well, silicone, glass, and steel toys, anyway. If you have a lot of toys, as your authors do, we recommend doing a full load just for them, using the pots and pans setting and very little soap. The heat and hot water will clean the devil right out of them. If you only have one or two, go ahead and throw them in the top rack with a regular load, then give them a rinse afterward to get rid of any leftover soap scum.

Another fun way to sterilize is with a good old-fashioned dildo boil! That's right, dig out your largest pot, fill it with water, and bring it to a boil. Then just throw in the dildos. In a few minutes, anything trying to hitch a ride on them will be well and thoroughly killed. Just remember to use tongs and oven mitts to retrieve your toys as many can retain a surprising amount of heat.

"If it's just for me, do I have to sterilize it?" you ask.

No, you really don't. Here's an occasion where soap and water can be perfectly sufficient even with toys made of more porous materials, because you aren't risking spreading bacteria or viruses to anyone else. However, we do not recommend jelly toys at all. As we'll get more into later, some jelly and PVC toys contain toxic phthalates.

Toy cleaner is also sold at every sex shop, but what most companies won't tell you is that this cleaner is very much like a household cleaner or disinfectant, and soap and water do the same job. It's also worth noting that some of the no-name toy cleaners may not be fully body-safe and there's no regulatory committee taking charge of this. There are some cleaning devices on the market that use UV lights and enclosed spaces to sanitize. These are pretty interesting, as we know that UV light will kill bacteria, viruses, and microbes. It won't, however, wipe off that poop. So, if you're going to clean that off anyway, why not just chuck the toy in the dishwasher?

One more way to sterilize is with rubbing alcohol or alcohol wipes. As a result of the COVID-19 pandemic, we likely all have a stash of this. Silicone toys especially deal just fine with being sprayed or rubbed with alcohol. We have a friend who used to spray down his metal toys and light them on fire. Dramatic? Yes. Awesome? Also, yes. Necessary? Probably not.

Safer Sex

The vastness of the safer sex discussion is a bit beyond the scope of this book, as really pegging is a pretty damned safe form of sex—after all, genitals never touch each other during this specific act. We are not, however, naive enough to believe that you're not going to include other kinds of fucking alongside pegging. Sex is, after all, a smorgasbord of delights. So, we're going to go into making your sex safer.

We recognize up front that many couples or pairings will be fluid bonded—as briefly mentioned earlier, this just means being willing to either put your fluids into another human or to receive theirs in you. Or both.

Philosophically, we subscribe to the idea of risk-aware sex, as we acknowledge that no form of sex is 100 percent safe. (And by *safe* we're referring here to the likelihood of adverse effects from sex including sexually transmitted infections, small humans, triggering anxiety, and we suppose…arguments?) By calling our approach "risk-aware sex," we're taking all of that as a given, and doing our best to understand our risks and do what we can to mitigate them to a decent extent. But, like skydiving, risk can come with reward. Sex is pretty rewarding.

Safer Sex Kits

We know what you're thinking. A casual skim over the next section and the following checklist feels like a level of preparation that no one needs. We get it, really. Even noted germophobic hypochondriac Cooper gets it. What it is, though, is an overview of a full-on "be prepared" kit that will get you by in any situation. Keep in mind that some of our readers are those weirdos (whom we love, and sometimes are) called swingers who go to full-on sex parties. There, it's not only important to be prepared for one situation, but many. But being prepared is also relevant if you're in the dating scene or cheating on your partner. (Which we, of course, discourage, but if you're going to cheat, the *least* you can do is protect your partner's sexual safety.)

Enough preamble. The following safer sex kit was built in a washroom supplies travel kit. Other great kit bases are shaving kits, first aid kits, or even computer accessory organizers. A trip to a certain online retailer will likely provide you with what you need to get started.

Condoms

Of course, right? As a sexual being, you should always carry condoms. If you enjoy the company of penises in any way, you should have condoms on you. Relying on someone else to provide a condom is a good way to get yourself into a situation where someone might try to coerce you to have sex without one due to lack of availability.

If you are the only penis wielder in the situation, you may stick with your own preferred condom size, but if you anticipate condoms may be needed in different sizes, you should probably carry both regular and large. You don't need to have an enormous penis to be well served by larger condoms, and it's worth trying multiple sizes to find your right fit. Seriously!

Since toys, no matter the size, don't have to worry about their blood supply being cut off by condoms, you don't need large ones for them, but we do recommend using condoms on toys as a matter of course.

Lastly, if you use condoms for blowjobs, first we applaud your safety initiative, and second, you may want to use a flavored condom. The note on this is that rarely do they come in non-latex, and rarely in any size but standard. If you don't use condoms for oral, there's really very little point to flavoring. But you do you.

Oral Barriers

Yep, the above section is not the last time we're going to talk about using barriers for oral sex. This is truly for those who are going above and beyond in their safety pursuits, and many opt not to. The nice thing about having barriers with you, however, is that you're prepared for any situation, rather than just your usual.

The classic example of an oral barrier is the dental dam. It's a small piece of latex designed to be placed over genitals and then licked through. Dental dams come in multiple sizes and flavors, and can be good in a pinch. But in general, dental dams kinda suck. They're often opaque and thicker than you'd like, not to mention rather small, with coverage that often amounts to *this* OR *that*.

Because of these many shortcomings, some people (Cooper included) have taken to carrying plastic wrap. Yes, just like the kind you use in the kitchen. As with our earlier "not doctors" disclaimers, we're going to hit you with a "not scientists" disclaimer here.

Is plastic wrap as safe as a dental dam? Probably?

Why can we only say probably? Well, because the FDA has never—and likely never will—approve plastic wrap for preventing the spread of STIs. Because why on earth would they ever do that? There's also a distinct lack of interest and funding for any sexuality research in our rather puritan society.

That said, many experiments have been done involving plastic wrap and what size molecules can penetrate it, and those molecules are all *way* smaller than the various viruses we're worried about being transmitted here—namely HPV and HSV (herpes simplex viruses)—so that allows for great confidence.

We will concede that oral sex is a fairly benign sexual activity when it comes to transmission, especially mouth to vulva, and are therefore comfortable with a number less than 99 percent for viral protection, even if we don't know what that number is. If you're using an oral barrier of any type, it's gonna be safer than not using one.

We will emphasize, though, that analingus *does* come with various potential bacterial issues. You can get non-STI transmission of things that you absolutely do not want. Which is why we do recommend that barrier for salad tossing.

Lube

Should lube really be considered a safer sex thing? Well, it does reduce friction, which reduces the possibility of skin abrasions and of compromising the integrity of your safer sex barriers, so we say yes.

The cornerstone of this kit is bringing whatever you might need for a given good time, and that certainly includes lube, because you don't want drugstore "lube" for your pegging encounters. Also, don't be tempted to get all creative with household things like olive oil or Crisco.

Some of your better lube companies will sell their products in packets that go nicely in safer sex kits. Check out the upcoming Best Tools for the Job section for more on lube.

Gloves

As mentioned earlier, gloves are wonderfully smooth accessories, and can really make for some awesome sex play and massages. They also keep lube off your hands, which is good because that stuff can get sticky after a while. On top of that, they are great for protecting both the glove wearer and the receiver from skin abrasions and hangnails, and really anything else going on with your hands.

Regardless of what you have in your safer sex kit, or how much it resembles the (to use a pun) anal level of this kit, the safer you are, the less you have to worry about, and the more pleasure you can have without devoting any portion of your brain's energy to "what if I die?!"

Build Your Safer Sex Kit

You may not need everything on this list, but it sure doesn't hurt! Some of the later things are just bonus care items. To house your supplies, shaving and makeup bags are great, as are travel bathroom kits.

To Buy To Pack

☐   ☐   Condoms (multiple sizes)

☐   ☐   Lube (silicone and water-based)

☐   ☐   Oral barriers (or plastic wrap)

☐   ☐   Gloves (multiple sizes)

☐   ☐   Wet wipes

☐   ☐   Packet of pain-relief meds

☐   ☐   Breath strips

☐   ☐   Mouthwash

What's in It for Me?

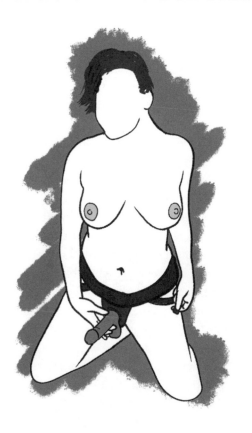

Beyond the Peg

When a woman straps that harness on and finds her-self with a dick between her legs, it's not only about prepping the receiver's ass to take it. She should take her time and flaunt that dick, using it in all the ways she's interested in. We have found that there are two major play opportunities that many never consider while using a harness and dildo.

First, the blowjob.

"But why would I want a blowjob?" you ask. "I can't even feel it."

While it's true you can't feel every lick and every suck, it's time to go to a mental place. Close your eyes for a moment and picture it, standing there, looking down at your huge cock jutting out from your pubis. Your partner kneeling before you, looking up at you with hunger in their eyes, maybe a bit of intimidation because of the size of your member. You reach out and slide your fingers in his hair, pulling him forward, and saying "I know it's pretty, but I didn't take it out for you to look at it—suck it, baby."

Perhaps that's a bit more than you're going for, but what we're trying to demonstrate is that a big part of all of this is mental anyway. The blowjob may not be as much about direct stimulation for you as for the mental role reversal, for the penis envy you may or may not have, for the domination or submission, for watching him just suck *your* cock.

It's not uncommon for women to get to relax into sex more a bit more than their male partners get to. We're not saying all women are pillow princesses who just "get fucked" and never do the fucking—any woman who's spent a few minutes on top knows that being the fucker can be strenuous work. But actually doing the thrusting is *hard*. It's exhausting and the first couple of times you peg, you may find that those muscles are sadly unprepared for that kind of workout.

Our advice: stretch before you peg! Before or after you put that harness and dildo on (after if you want to give your partner a fun show) be sure to stand upright, raise your hands above your head and stretch up to the ceiling, then bend at your waist, and try to touch your toes or the floor. Don't push yourself past where it is comfortable to go. Do pelvic circles: engage your core muscles and thrust your hips from the right side to the back, to the left side, back to the front until it becomes a fluid circular motion. Do them clockwise for a few rotations, then counterclockwise. Twist your top half from side to side while keeping your hips straight to stretch out your spine a bit.

Take water breaks as needed. Just like any exercise, you want to make sure you're hydrated. This is especially important if alcohol or marijuana is involved as both can make one feel dehydrated or cotton-mouthed. We want all orifices to be well lubricated when it comes to pegging!

Feel free to change up the position. Sometimes the pegger can have a limb fall asleep, become strained from being in one position too long, get a charley horse or muscle spasm, or just become super uncomfortable in a certain position. Refer to the position guide if you need ideas; try out a few to see what works best for your bodies and flexibility levels.

Being the thruster can be a lot of work, so if for no other reason, use pegging as your next fun workout challenge. A pleasurable night of pegging usually gives the pegger morning-after abs that feel like they spent the whole night laughing or doing crunches— that hurts-so-good kind of muscle pain.

Tit for Tat

Sometimes the pegging conversation is initiated in a hetero relationship because the man wants to have anal sex with his partner and she responds with something along the lines of, "If you do it, I'll do it." This might not be the healthiest way to get into anal play, but if both parties are interested, game, and enthusiastically consenting to the play on both sides, it can be nice to explore together simultaneously. Since a lot of the anal sex basics that we cover here are unisex and universal, exploring anal play at the same time can be a fun experiment.

A lot of menfolk are super excited about anal sex and think that, like any average porn star, they can just go to town with no prep or even lube. Being on the other side of that equation will give any man some much-needed knowledge about what the receiver of their dick will probably go through. Understanding the need for communication, lubrication, and patience is essential for anal play for both men and women.

On the flip side, women experiencing receiving anal sex will have more insight into what care and communication needs to be had before strapping on and diving in.

Oftentimes, both parties will find that slow and steady wins the race, not the pile-driver pounding that we so often see in porn. A fun scene to plan for might be to start off with pegging, but not to fruition, and end with the pegger receiving anal sex, so both sides get in on the fun. Throw in a nice massage before and between acts for both parties to limber up, and you have yourself a fine evening of sensual, uni-sexual, anal experience.

Mistress Peggy

Not everyone is into BDSM, topping, dominance, or control, but if you are one of those kinky people, pegging can be a great way to turn the tables on a partner who may always feel the need to be on top, be in control, or play the part of the "fucker."

Kink is sometimes the goal, but interestingly, this is how Andre Shakti answered when we asked, "What's one thing you think the world should know about pegging?"

She replied, "That pegging can be sensual. I think a lot of times, pegging gets lumped into the kink and BDSM categories, and while there can be kinky elements to pegging, while there can of course be power play, while there can be roleplay involved or there can be other, you know, kink-related or fetish-related activities involved.

"That pegging can be just as sensual and loving and connective as any other kind of sexual experience. I would say half of the clients that I get as a dominatrix, they specially request more of a heavy femme Dom BDSM scene, where there's humiliation involved, there's maybe some bondage incorporated, maybe some roleplay. You know, they're calling me honorifics, that kind of thing, while I'm doing the pegging. And that's largely because I think that still most of the pegging porn that's out there is very kind of strict, like, women taking charge in a very leather-clad and, you know, procedural-related way. And to a point where, it's almost stripped the sexuality from the act like, in my opinion, it's almost stripped the intimacy from the act. And hey, if you are into that role, rigid, BDSM pegging as power play, that's completely valid and legitimate and hot, right?

"I think that a lot of folks assume or, from my experience, a lot of men assume there has to be some of that hard dynamic when it comes to pegging and in reality, I also, again, half the time, get very, very, shy requests for a more sensual experience. You know, can you pretend like you're my girlfriend and you're doing this with me? And I think that is, you know, just as powerful, if not more powerful, of something to ask for an experience than just jumping to the conclusion that pegging has to like, inherently be kinky.

"I know for a lot of people the idea of pegging is just as kinky as the idea of, you know, choking somebody consensually during sex or even doing like consensual non-consent play, but I don't know, I just don't see it like that."

Pegging can be a great way to experiment with aspects of BDSM, if both of you are game. Pegging is one of those dynamic sexual acts where one can top or bottom from both sides of the harness. A person being pegged could be doing the directing, giving demands to the pegger on how to perform, how to move, what to do, or they could be the one submitting and relinquishing control entirely.

Depending on how intense your play gets, or the power dynamic you use, you may want to establish some safewords beforehand. It's a bit outside our scope, but the only real rule with safewords is that whatever you use wouldn't be something you would normally say during sex. If items like gags will be used and prevent good verbal communication, there are physical nonverbal safe actions like snapping fingers, dropping something the bottom is instructed to hold during the scene, blinking rapidly, or shaking your head. Whatever the word or action you choose, make it absolutely clear beforehand and respect it immediately if used. A safeword means the end of the scene, a check-in, and potentially the start of some much-needed aftercare. A healthy kink dynamic is one where both parties feel comfortable saying their safeword if the situation calls for it.

Communication in kink play is always key, whether it's aloud or body language cues. Be very mindful of your partner's body as well as your own. Pegging can be taxing on both sides and caring for your partner, as well as self-care, is important.

Fucking Pleasure

Folks in our pegging class like to ask what pleasure women get out of pegging if the dick isn't part of their actual body and it's devoid of the nerve endings needed to get off. There are a lot of factors to "getting off" when it comes to our bodies, so let's start at the most obvious. For 30 to 80 percent of women in the world (the studies vary dramatically), orgasming is only possible with clitoral stimulation, and where does the dildo on a harness usually rest? Yep, right on the clit.

Many harnessable dildos vibrate, and the bullet or motor of the dildo is often set into the base, right up against the clit of the pegger. This may be overwhelming for some people, so be wary of over-using the vibration modes. Vibration is also a great way to add some natural numbing to the ass when getting ready to peg, or just added sensation to a very sensitive area, but it can also numb the pegger, which is less ideal. Your sensitivity to vibration will vary, so find a vibrating dildo with a bullet that you can switch out for low or high intensity if you want to experiment with vibration during pegging.

Along with clitoral stimulation, there are a number of pegging toys (which we'll get more into in the Best Tools for the Job section) that are dual-ended and insertable, meaning there's a part that inserts into the vagina and another that juts out to penetrate a partner. Some of these vibrate, some are curved up to hit the G-spot, and some are just bulbs for holding onto as a harnessless dildo. The curved insertable toys are particularly nice for pegging as each thrust pulls gently against the G-spot and can be an amazing way of each partner receiving an internal orgasm together.

Some women who have experience with squirting orgasms have found that the sensations involved in pegging can lead them to an ejaculatory orgasm, giving the sensation of coming "inside" the peggee.

Aside from the purely physical aspects that make fucking pleasurable, there are also the mental aspects. Like filling your partner's most sensitive holes, giving them an amazing body-shaking orgasm, fulfilling a desire of yours or theirs that is new and exciting, connecting sexually on an extremely intimate level, and coming to new understandings of trust and vulnerability within your relationship.

What If They Don't Come?

Sometimes pegging is going to be your partner's ultimate fantasy but it still won't get them *there*. This is totally normal and doesn't mean you are doing anything wrong. We delved into the anatomy of the prostate orgasm earlier, but just wanted to give y'all a reminder: sometimes they won't come from pegging alone and that's okay.

Just as most women won't (or can't) come from penetration alone, putting pressure on any person to come in just one way or another actually makes it *much* harder to come that way.

Pegging can already be rather intense, and when dealing with a new experience and new sensations, your body can react in all sorts of ways. Sometimes that's coming super quickly in a tidal wave of teenage-like endorphins, and sometimes it's shutting down the come-function and just riding out the waves of pleasure. With practice, a couple will figure out what works for them.

If the person being pegged does not come from pegging alone, but they still want to come, switch things up and ask if they would like to come another way. Would a toy help, would they like a handjob or blowjob, would they like to switch to PIV sex? Sex has many options and you can always stop during one act if it's not working out and switch to something else. We're not saying give up necessarily, but there are times when you're driving and miss your exit and there's just no easy way to go backwards on the highway. Sometimes you just need to find another way home.

There's also the idea of trying to have non-goal-orientated sex where the end point isn't orgasm per se, but just having fun. This can be hard for many of us because we've been conditioned to think the end of sex is always coming, for one or both (or all) parties involved, but it's worthwhile experimenting with sex where fun is the goal and orgasm is a potential bonus. Hooray if you get there, but it's okay if you don't.

Best Tools for the Job

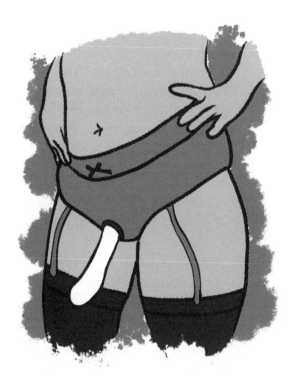

Where to Buy

Buying from a progressive, sex-positive, adult toy store has a *lot* of benefits, but one of the main ones is that you can usually hold the items in your hands before you buy. Sometimes you can even try harnesses on (over your clothes) to see how they would feel. We can't stress enough how important it is to keep these businesses afloat—buying through big box brands or evil corporations that will not be named is slowly killing them. Support your local sex shop and spend your money where it really counts. When searching for a brick-and-mortar store near you, some good search terms are "feminist sex toy store" or "female-owned and operated sex toy store." Many of these brick-and-mortar stores also have online shops, including Lyndzi's home base shop, The Tool Shed. Shevibe, Good Vibrations, and The Pleasure Chest are also among the best options.

Harnesses/Straps

Let's start with the wearable pegging gear before we get into the fleshy bits. Harnesses are sometimes an afterthought, but they are just as important as the tool you put into them. They range from comfortable cotton boxer shorts to hot pink sparkly studded vinyl straps. They're incredibly customizable and have almost as much variety as the toys themselves. There are some key factors you will want to consider when going into a harness purchase, or, as we like to say, harness *investment*.

Other things to consider: How big are the hips that will be wearing this harness? What level of comfort does the wearer want? Do you prefer cotton, leather, elastic, nylon, vinyl, latex, velvet, rubber, spandex, or another specific material? Are you or your partner allergic to any materials or against wearing animal products like leather? Do you want to wear the harness like a pair of underwear, like a jock strap, or like a G-string? Do you want to be able to throw it in the washer and dryer? How much are you willing to spend? Do you like the look and feel of buckles, velcro, or D-rings? How big will the toy that you plan to use be, and therefore how wide will the O-ring on the harness need to be? Once you've pondered these questions, here are some options to look into.

Underwear-Style Harnesses

Underwear-style harnesses, made popular by the brand RodeoH, are usually made of a soft cotton material, and there are no straps, buckles, or metal rings to deal with. They are designed in many different styles, including ones that look like a pair of boxers, briefs, or fancy lace panties. They usually have some extra inner pockets for vibrating bullets, which is a fun feature.

These are tops in comfort level, but may not be the best in effectiveness depending on the toy you pair with it. The elastic waistband, if not properly fitted to the wearer's body, can be droopy and stretch if the toy is too heavy. Most pegging toys are rather light, but double-ended toys (that are also insertable for the wearer) tend to be on the heavier side. The pocket flap inside most underwear-style harnesses can usually be pulled down so a double-ended toy can be used, though it can be a little awkward and pull the top of the underwear down, making it feel less stable. That flap can also be worn up with a flat-based toy so the toy material doesn't have to touch their skin at all if they don't want it to.

The O-rings in these harnesses are sewn in, so they are not adjustable. They can usually hold up to a two-inch toy, but nothing girthier than that. The cotton sides of the opening can often make it difficult to push a silicone toy through, but a trick we have found is placing a small plastic bag over the toy, slipping it through the O-ring, then pulling the bag off. Choosing a toy with a large base can also make these awkward to wear. If your toy has huge testicles and a flared suction-cup base, it's not going to be flush against your body and will pull the underwear forward quite a bit.

This option is usually mid-range in price ($40–$60) but often not as long-lasting as other harnesses. They are machine washable, though we have found if you hand-wash them and let them air dry, they last a lot longer. They are usually sized to a three- to five-inch range, so sizing correctly is essential. Too loose and the undies will slip down with the weight of the toy, too tight and you won't be able to get them over your hips.

Strappy Straps

This style is usually the most common entry-level harness. They are super adjustable, as they usually include long nylon or leather straps. The way to get these harnesses on is to loosen the straps, step into them, then tighten the straps to your hips, legs, and around your butt. Depending on the harness, there may be multiple straps to tighten.

There are a few different types of this basic style, most common being the two-leg-strap jock style or the one-strap G-string style. What's nice about these harnesses is that the O-ring can usually be taken out and replaced with a different size or different material ring (rings can be made of stretchy rubber or solid metal).

Material is a factor that will play into this style and affect the price quite a bit. Leather is long-lasting, but expensive. Nylon can be a little abrasive on the skin, but it's super cheap. D-rings, which are usually on nylon strap harnesses to adjust the size, can slip and have to be readjusted occasionally, but buckles, which are usually on leather harnesses, will keep to the size you set them at, much like a belt.

There are strap harnesses where the O-ring is connected to the waistband and others where it is off-set and drops lower than the waistband. We prefer the latter as we don't know many folks with vulvae directly under their belly buttons. If you want the toy's base to hit at the lower belly/waist area, then the option with the higher O-ring might work just fine.

Straps make these harnesses adjustable, and they can therefore fit multiple partners or still be used if your body changes. Prices vary from super-cheap nylon strap harnesses in the $20–$40 range to sophisticated, made-in-America, top-of-the-line spandex harnesses that will run easily over $100.

Fashion Harnesses
We have seen some fancy harnesses on display at various sex toy stores and sex-positive conferences. Folks can get really elaborate with harness designs. There are crushed red velvet corset-backed harnesses that look like a Victorian kinkster's wet dream, and spike-studded vegan-leather harnesses that look like the wearer could kick your ass while making you a matcha tea. We've seen harnesses made of chain, duct tape, as part of a latex catsuit, incorporated into an elaborate shibari rope tie, made from recycled bicycle

tires, bejeweled with rhinestones, in every color of the rainbow, and there are more unique designs being created every day. The sky's the limit for showing off your style with your harness.

A note here, though—sometimes things designed to look good aren't designed with functionality in mind. For example, if those rhinestones are in a spot where they might pound into your partner's tender bits, they might not be so much fun!

Dildos

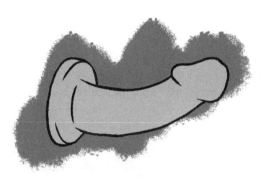

Often when choosing a new toy, the number of options can be overwhelming. Depending on where you're buying, you can be surrounded by dicks of every shape, size, and color. You can easily find yourself scrolling a website for pages and pages trying to figure out what seven inches really even looks like. In a sex-positive toy store setting, you're usually allowed to pick up and handle a toy before you buy it. This is specifically so you know the feel, weight, firmness, and flexibility of the product. We will often joke that "the wand chooses the wizard," as the one that feels just right for you will usually become quite clear after handling a few.

There are a few key things to consider when finding the right tool for the job: toy material, realism, length, girth, firmness, and shape.

Toy Material

Toy material is an important consideration, though we'd like to make it super simple for you. As we mentioned earlier, our recommendation is 100 percent silicone. Always go with silicone. There are other materials out there that may be cheaper, softer, or more fun looking, but when it comes to a harnessable dildo for pegging, silicone is your best choice. Medical-grade silicone is body-safe, hypoallergenic, non-porous, easy to clean, can be sterilized, often very long-lasting, and durable.

The reason we rail against using toys made of plastic, elastomer, rubber, vinyl, Realskin, jelly, or anything other than silicone is that these materials are not regulated in any way and the chemicals that toy manufacturers add to these materials to make them soft and squishy can leach out onto *or into* you. When we talk about sexy scenes, chemical burns are kind of the opposite of the scene we want to set.

Purchase your silicone toys from reputable retailers and companies, not conglomerate websites, which often sell knockoffs. These conglomerate sites are also where folks can resell their used toys (yes, people can and do actually do that, so be careful!).

We know that cheap toys are just that, cheaper, and we understand that not everyone can afford the best of the best in high-end toys. Still, we urge you to consider your sexy tools an investment worth spending a bit on. You and your partner's safety, health, and genitals are worth it.

"But if it's cheap, why does it matter what it's made of?" you ask.

Much as we applaud your frugality in these uncertain economic times, jelly dildos have fallen dramatically out of favor for two major reasons. One, they are porous. This means that, like an English Muffin, they're full of all sorts of nooks and crannies for literally anything and everything to hang out in even after washing. That's a big eew from us. And two...well...they fucking melt! And we don't just mean from heat.

If you Google "jelly dildo melt" and click on almost any of the results, you'll see exactly why. If you store these dildos together, they melt and meld into some Lovecraftian monstrosity in a shockingly short amount of time. And even if they're not stored with any others, if you leave one in the bottom of your bedside drawer for too long, when you pull it out it'll be misshapen and flat on one side and *may* have begun to fuse with the bottom of your drawer.

More modern dildos do still come in this awful jelly, but also come in proprietary blends like Realskin, or elastomer. These are better than jelly without question, but most still have pores and are thus petri dishes.

Realism

Some peggers want their dildo to feel like an extension of themselves and gravitate to a super-realistic-looking cock. Some peggees, however, may not feel comfortable with something that looks realistic and prefer something in a wild color and/or a smooth finish with no realistic-looking penis "head." Your mileage may vary, but sometimes these are very strong feelings, so you should communicate with one another before you buy or, better yet, go shopping for all your pegging needs together. The only real difference in feel or useability between realistic and non-realistic is going to be the coronal ridge or head of the toy. As the ridge gives a slight hook to the end of the toy, it can be used to press up against and massage the prostate.

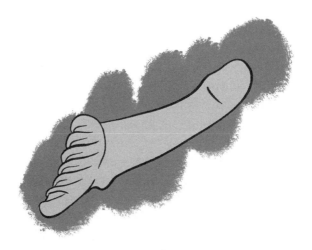

Length

As fun as sword fighting with any dildo can be (while wearing it, even more so), length is an important factor. A silicone dildo that's too long can be floppy and hard to control, so thrusting can be difficult and unreliable. However, a dildo that is too short may slip out during penetration, which can be quite the surprise and an uncomfortable sensation during anal sex. Body size is a good determining factor when it comes to considering dildo size. If the pegger has a bigger belly, or if they want to hold onto the base of the toy, longer is better. If the intention is to hit the prostate, explore to find how far into the anal canal the perfect spot is, then use that to determine a good toy length, as the head of the toy should hit at right that length.

Girth

When it comes to anal sex, we like to joke that the end of your ass is your mouth. Meaning that toys can be pretty long, but girth is really what counts. The anal sphincter has to stretch during anal sex on any body, and every body has a different threshold of how much is comfortable. Stretching the sphincter is very common in prepping for anal play. Using toys like butt plugs that gradually increase in size can help the body get used to more girth. We always suggest starting small, even just with fingers or finger-sized anal-safe toys, to get your body used to the sensation. Then, when you feel comfortable, work your way up to bigger girth sizes. Even veteran anal porn superstars have to prep for big anal scenes, sometimes using gradually bigger toys throughout the day before a shoot.

It's a common concern and myth that someone can become stretched out or never return to normal. While stretching and loosening the butthole is something that does happen, it's typically only achieved for a short amount of time, maybe a few hours max. Except in extreme cases, someone being stretched open shouldn't worry about remaining that way.

Firmness

Firmness and function go hand in hand, but the level of firmness can also affect the level of comfort for the receiver. Function-wise, softer toys may be floppy and too bendy to be useful, whereas a stiff toy is going to go in the direction you poke it. A softer toy may have more give and the squish factor may make it seem more realistic and comfortable, but will most likely require more lubrication. Prostates generally respond well to firm stimulation, so toy materials like firm silicone, glass, and stainless steel make for good prostate toys. As we've discussed, strap-on play isn't really conducive to glass or stainless steel toys, so peggers would do well to find a firm silicone toy for the easiest use.

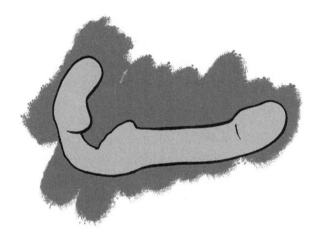

Shape

There are many shape options for strap-on toys. There are toys that replicate the shape of a human penis right down to tiny veins and hair follicles, and others made to the shape of an anatomically correct horse cock or a mythical dragon dick in marbled galaxy sparkle colors. The possibilities are endless and with so many independent crafter silicone makers out there, customization is at a peak. Of the more basic, run-of-the-mill variety of dildos out there, the shape factors you want to keep in mind are flat, suction-cup, or insertable base, and type of curve.

The myth of the "strapless dildo" is pervasive and many toy companies claim to have found the key to an insertable/double-ended toy that can be worn by a person in their vagina or anus, and for it to jut outward from their body like a biological cock without the aid of a harness or belt of any kind. The problem often falls on the weight of said toy and the pelvic floor muscles of said wearer. Many silicone toys are quite dense and heavy. Unless you have Kegel muscles of steel, it's going to be tough to keep a silicone "erection" upright and not have it pop out in the heat of the moment. Also, orgasms, it turns out, are by definition contractions of the pelvic floor muscles, which will force a toy out unless strapped on tight. If the wearer assumes or anticipates that they may have an orgasm while pegging (hey, here's hoping!), then they may want to brace the toy with something to make sure they don't shoot it out right at the climax of their sexy time.

All of this isn't to cancel double-ended insertable dildos. In fact, just the opposite—they really are a lot of fun! If the wearer of an insertable dildo has a G-spot, the toy pushes right up against it, making pegging especially fun for the penetrator. It can give the pegger a sense of fullness and of being fucked as well as doing the fucking. They just need to stabilize it in some way. Sometimes that can be as simple as wearing a tight pair of boxer briefs with an opening in the front for the toy or a harness made out of rope or a silky tie, or as complex as a lacy crotchless underwear harness with garters and sequined trim.

You do you, but if you have a double-ended dildo, do it with stability.

Curved toys are great for G-spot and prostate play, depending on the position. You can refer to the pegging position guide for some ideas as to which positions do best for curved toys if a good cock bend is your cup of tea.

Lubes

We love lube! It's one of science's greatest gifts to vagina- and anus-havers alike. Unlike the vagina, the anus does not self-lubricate, so when engaging in any kind of anal play, lube is absolutely necessary. There are a lot of types out there to consider though, so let's get into it.

Water-Based

Water-based lubes are great all around. They're body-safe; feel more natural; are compatible with condoms, dental dams, and gloves of any type; and work well with toys of any material.

Water-based lubes can be eaten safely. We don't recommend tucking in with a bowl of lube, but just wanted to note that there's no need to be afraid of water-based lube getting in your mouth. There are some nicely flavored ones on the market for exactly this purpose.

The only downside is, much like natural lubrication (which is also water-based), these lubes are not as long-lasting as other types. Water-based lubes will soak into the skin with enough friction or over enough time. To combat this, most folks just reapply as needed. Some companies now make thicker water-based lubes that feel like gel and offer more of a cushion, which can be quite nice with anal play as they are longer-lasting.

Silicone-Based

Silicone lube is great for body-to-body sex but toy users may want to be careful when using silicone on a silicone toy. There's been some debate on how much damage silicone lube does to 100 percent silicone toys, but, just in case, we always test the toy out (apply some lube to a small spot on the bottom of the toy and leave it overnight to see what happens). Or better yet, cover the silicone toy in a condom before applying lube to prevent potentially ruining your favorite toy. The damage in question has ranged from nothing at all to the surface of the toy starting to flake off (like dry skin after a sunburn), to the toy looking like it was melted a bit. Your mileage may vary, especially taking into consideration the quality of the silicone used to make the toy. Some silicone toys can be quite pricy, and we would never want you to harm your favorite cock, so be careful!

An awesome thing about silicone lube is it is *very* slippery. A concerning thing about silicone lube is that it is *very* slippery. Unlike water-based lubricants, silicone won't soak into your skin, even with friction or water. Oftentimes after putting silicone lube on our hands and washing them with soap, they'll still feel a little slippery. This long-lasting nature is a gift and a curse. It's great during sex. A little silicone lube goes a long way and sex with it is just a slippery, lovely mess. It can leave a slippery residue that has to be cleaned off and can even stain sheets if spilled, dribbled, or wiped on them.

Like water-based lubes, silicone is safe with condoms, dental dams, and gloves, but as stated previously, it can harm silicone toys. When it comes to non-silicone toys, like porous elastomer toys (usually cheap jelly dongs or masturbation sleeves), it won't necessarily harm them, but silicone can get into the pores of the toy, be hard to clean off, and stay slippery seemingly forever. When it comes to glass, stainless steel, or hard plastic toys, silicone lube is totally fine to use—just be warned, it makes things super slippery, and a glass or stainless steel toy slipping out and onto the floor (or worse, a toe!), is a real mood-killer.

Overall, silicone lube is great for anal play because you want the most slip and least friction on the anus as possible.

Hybrid

Any lube that calls itself a hybrid usually just means it's a blend of water and silicone. Oftentimes, though not always, it's mostly water-based so fully toy-safe, but the added silicone makes it a little extra slippery. When it comes to pegging play, we almost always point folks in the direction of the hybrid lubes for this reason. Toy-safe and slippery—best of both worlds!

Oil-Based

Oil-based lubes are often marketed as just masturbation lubes, but some folks do use oil-based products as lubricants during sex (think coconut oil, olive oil, massage oil, Crisco, etc.), so we're going to go over both oil-based lubes and oil products that you could *technically* use for sex.

First off, oil of any kind is not safe with latex condoms or gloves. Oil can cause them to break down, and can very easily and quickly cause holes and rips, making these safer sex items no longer safer at all.

Oil is also not vagina-friendly as it doesn't get flushed out of the vagina easily and can harbor bacteria if left inside, sometimes leading to pesky things like UTIs or yeast infections. Oil is fine for anal play. Many people swear by coconut oil especially. Like silicone, oil is super slippery and long-lasting. Silicone toys are also compatible with oil products, but be sure the toy is 100 percent silicone, as oil can break down softer-material toys like elastomer masturbation sleeves.

You'll have to see what your bodies tolerate or like, as everybody is different. What we can say is that using food oils is definitely in the "iffier" direction in terms of safety, so we will always recommend using products that are specifically designed for lubricating dicks or butts or vaginas.

A Warning on Numbing Lubes

As discussed in the Safety and Comfort chapter, anal sex shouldn't need a numbing agent. There are many natural ways to relax the sphincter muscles without losing sensation. Numbing products can be potentially dangerous and make things less fun for both the user and their partner. If you're tempted to go out and buy yourself a bottle of numbing lube, head on back to the Safety and Comfort section and reread it to ease your mind. Anal sex should be fun, not painful, and usually lubrication and communication are the answer, not deadening our body's pain receptors.

Positioning Aids

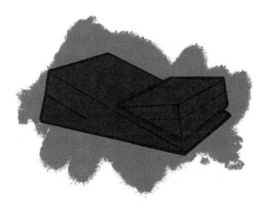

Initially designed for older folks with hip and mobility issues, positioning aids started to become super popular sellers in the early 2000s for a younger demographic who quickly realized how much fun they can be when added to sexual activities.

These products are usually shaped like a wedge, but come in a bunch of different shapes and styles. Some have holes for vibrators or masturbation sleeves, some are rounded with a dramatic curved side to be able to rock back and forth on, or for a person to drape over, and some now even come with bondage accessories sewn on for a kinky play element. These pillows are extra-firm, so they don't deflate during sex. If you've ever tried to just use a pillow or two underneath your hips during sex, you may have discovered they get squished down relatively fast and are rendered useless after a few minutes. Wedges like the ones made by Liberator (an American-owned company known for their sexy positioning aids), are constructed with super-firm foam that doesn't deflate under pressure, yet is still soft enough to not be uncomfortable.

Aids are particularly nice for folks with joint pain and can help prevent sore wrists, elbows, knees, and hips by elevating the sensitive bits. They often include removable covers for easy washing.

Fancy pillows aren't always necessary to get the perfect angle though. If you do have some firm pillows of your own, you can try them out. The deflation problem always depends on the firmness of said pillow, so experimentation may be needed. There is also a product called a doggy strap (because it's used during the doggy-style position), which is simply a padded strap of nylon to be used around the hips of the person on all fours. The ends of the straps have handles for the person behind, and it allows extra leverage for that person to pull their partner toward them without grabbing onto the love handle area.

There are a lot of creative ways to get into that perfect position to hit just the right spot, but understand that your body has limits and purchasing (or DIY-ing) something to help you get there comfortably is always better than hurting yourself or your partner. Be careful with your bodies, folks—you only get one.

The Giving Revolution

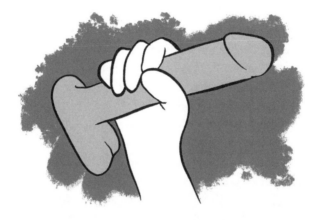

"Raise your glasses to the future!" we tell you, leaning back in our chairs. The night has grown old, and the drinks are little but water at the bottom of a glass. We, Cooper and Lyndzi, share a knowing glance because we've passed it along, and what better gift can people give than the sharing of pleasure?

As you leave the patio, you have so much to talk about, to think about. Maybe one of you is already online making equipment purchases while the other weighs in as they drive. Maybe tonight you take your first steps, first fumbling fingers in butts. Maybe all we've done is give your curiosity something to chew on. Whatever the case, you're leaving tonight with permission that wasn't ours to give you, but was yours to give yourself—permission to explore.

And thus, we leave the clumsy second-person prose behind in favor of reflecting on what a gift that is. This exploration in this book was primarily directed in that whole butthole region, but we'd like to leave you with a far more holistic idea.

We began this book by telling you that pegging is an anomaly in the sex-act world, because of how specific it is. And now we want to flip that idea on its head. There's ultimately no need for the gendering of pegging, and there's no need to differentiate it from any other type of anal sex.

So, why did we?

Well, that's a simple question with a complex answer. Conceptual abstracts are just that: abstract. We could write a book about anal sex, but you know who probably wouldn't read it? People who have very specific ideas about what anal sex is. And what is it? By and large, like almost every other precon-ception about sex, it's a gendered concept. And even worse, it's usually a homophobic gendered concept. Something only "those" men do. We all know that this isn't true, because so many of the people who believe it will think nothing of a man penetrating his wife or girlfriend anally. That doesn't count as gay, of course.

Ultimately anal sex can be scary, regardless of age, experience, or gender, if you've not had much experience receiving it. A huge swath of the population only has experience giving, being the thruster, being the penetrator—be it with fingers, with dicks, with tongues. Being the top, the pitcher. It's funny how we can let our identities get wrapped up in such concepts.

It's not exclusive to that, of course—the spectrums of sexuality/sexual identity/sexual expression are full of varying degrees of overlapping labels. Some are important, some are superfluous. And we're not going to sit here and tell you which is which. Because we can't.

Labels don't matter until they matter to you. For good or bad. And if you perceive yourself as a top, or pegger, or pitcher, or penetrator, and that's "who you are," well, that's fine. Everybody should be able to identify themselves however they want. Cooper could go on and on about how many LGBTQIA+ people have mentioned their discomfort with the label he applies to himself: queer.

Let's circle back to one of those terms, one of the terms that people who put appendages into others tend to use: giver. There are plenty of ways that this term could be interpreted in an icky way. The most ostensibly difficult version is that it's about a man giving a woman the gift of his seed. Yuck. We encourage you to think about it differently. You're probably mumbling "Thanks for putting that interpretation in our head before telling us not to think about it that way." Our bad.

Giver. The giver of a gift. What is the gift if not (bleh) seed? The phallus? The gift is, hopefully, giving the receiver what they desire.

Consent to penetrate can be an incredibly wrought concept. And that's ultimately what this all is. As the peggee, we're asking for the pegger to put something inside us. We're asking to receive them. We're asking to host them. And that's incredibly intimate.

There's the temptation when writing content like this to talk about the world as we wish it was. That world wouldn't call pegging a role reversal because it wouldn't need to. There wouldn't be the traditional roles of the penetrator and penetratee because sexual encounters would be about what's happening that specific time, rather than every time before and every time until the last time. (Got dark there.)

Something that the straight community could learn from the LGBTQIA+ community is the expansion of their sexual ideas leading to vastly more communication. Because the LGBTQIA+ community often doesn't subscribe to the "man putting something inside a woman" traditional planning of a sexual encounter, it means that sexual encounters have to be discussed beforehand.

It's easy, especially in long-term relationships, to see your sex as a repeating act. There's nothing wrong with this, of course. If you and your partner desire to have sex in the missionary position every time and you both enjoy it, good on you. But it's the part about "both enjoy it" that is essential there. Too often we allow our sex to fall into routines like anything else in our lives. If we didn't, there wouldn't be a cottage industry of "spice up your love life" books. Or this one, we guess.

Routine isn't bad. Let's get that out of the way. It's simply routine. Same isn't bad, it's simply same.

In talking to people all over the country and around the world, one thing we've seen time and time again is that one partner may be perfectly happy with routine while the other has an itch. That fabled seven-year itch of yore that often led to affairs. But behind that is often the desire for something different. The desire for *not* routine. So many of us in monogamous relationships think that the only thing that can provide difference is a new person. Because we think we're set. We're stuck. Not in the relationship, but in our perception of that relationship. And the simple act of communication is terrifying.

What we desire more than anything else for you, the reader, is for this book to start a conversation.

Whether that conversation leads to pegging or not is inconsequential to us. (Though, we hope that it does.) The most important thing any one of us can do for our sex life is to talk about it, interrogate it, explore it. Do we like the things we like because they're awesome (it's definitely possible they are) or because we feel we're supposed to like them?

The world has done an unfair number on us all, filling us with insidious opinions and ideas about our sexuality and others. And the healthiest thing we can all do about that is to strive to unlearn them.

When you open up and discuss your desires, your curiosities, and your explorations with a partner or playmate, it unlocks doors, and you're no longer sticking yourself with Monty Hall's insistence of "door number one."

While there are many ways to examine the necessity of the term pegging, we see it as one of those many other doors. Pegging as a concept isn't the end, because anyone who enjoys pegging tends to enjoy other types of anal exploration and play, and they tend not to associate the idea of anal sex with any specific group or preconception. This is progress.

That doorway marked pegging could be simply the latest exploration in a long life of exploration, or could mark your first forays outside simple conceptions of sex. Regardless of where you are on that spectrum, passing through the pegging doorway doesn't mean you stop there, but instead leads you to many other doors, other explorations you can choose to take or leave be.

Our willingness to explore, to converse, to learn, and to grow and change are the very foundations of a happy and satisfied life. And these things are without question the best things we can do as humans. Obviously, our purview with this book is about sexual exploration, learning, growing, and changing, but the idea is also true about how you choose to see the world.

The best version of you is one that is always growing and changing and learning. So, with us enthusiastically cheering you on, bend over to let in the new.

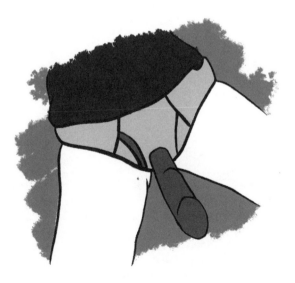

Index

Page numbers in *italics* indicate illustrations.

Also from Thornapple Press

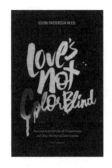

Love's Not Color Blind: Race and Representation in Polyamorous and Other Alternative Communities
Kevin A. Patterson, with a foreword by Ruby Bouie Johnson

"Kevin does amazing work both centering the voices of people of color and educating white folks on privilege. His words will positively influence polyamorous communities for years to come."
— Rebecca Hiles, The Frisky Fairy

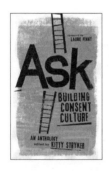

Ask: Building Consent Culture
Edited by Kitty Stryker, with a foreword by Laurie Penny

"There are certain conversations that deepen how you think; positively impact how you act; expand your view and understanding of the world, and forever alter how you approach it. This book is full of them. Make room for it—then spread the word."
— Alix Fox, journalist, sex educator and ambassador for the Brook sexual wellbeing charity

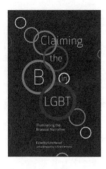

**Claiming the B in LGBT:
Illuminating the Bisexual Narrative**
Edited by Kate Harrad, with a
foreword by H. Sharif Williams

"With bisexuality becoming ever
more visible in mainstream culture,
this book is essential reading for bi
people and would-be allies, within
the LGBT community and beyond."
—Louise Carolin, deputy editor,
DIVA magazine

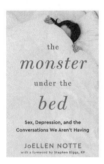

**The Monster Under the Bed:
Sex, Depression, and the
Conversations We Aren't Having**
JoEllen Notte, with a foreword
by Stephen Biggs, RP

"JoEllen dared to speak about a topic
no one else would and has changed
the way we think about sex and
depression. Her work is, quite simply,
invaluable."
—Tristan Taormino, sex educator,
host of Sex Out Loud Radio, and
author of *Opening Up*